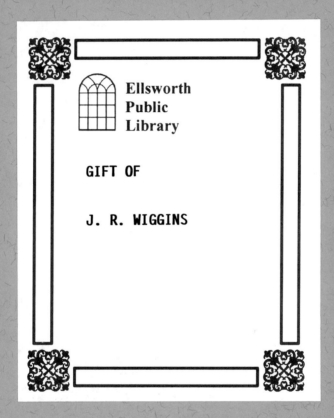
MW01042356

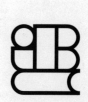

Crossing Boundaries

Love & Russ
from Bis

Seymour B. Sarason
Elizabeth M. Lorentz

Crossing Boundaries

Collaboration, Coordination, and the Redefinition of Resources

Jossey-Bass Publishers • San Francisco

Chapter Five excerpt by George Albee reprinted with permission of *Country Journal*, Cowles Enthusiast Media, 4 High Ridge Park, Stamford, CT 06905.

Chapter Six excerpt from "One on One" by Wendy Watriss, *The Texas Observer*, November 22, 1990. Reprinted with permission.

Epilogue excerpts by Manabu Sato reprinted from *Issues and Problems of Teacher Education*, Howard B. Leavitt, Ed. Copyright © 1992 by Greenwood Press. Reproduced with permission of Greenwood Publishing Group, Inc., Westport, CT.

For sales outside the United States, please contact your local Simon & Schuster International office.

Jossey-Bass Web address: http://www.josseybass.com

 Manufactured in the United States of America on Lyons Falls Turin Book. This paper is acid-free and 100 percent totally chlorine-free.

Library of Congress Cataloging-in-Publication Data

Sarason, Seymour B., date.
    Crossing boundaries : collaboration, coordination, and the redefinition of resources / Seymour B. Sarason, Elizabeth M. Lorentz. — 1st ed.
        p.   cm.
    Includes bibliographical references and index.
    ISBN 0-7879-1069-4 (cloth : acid-free paper)
    1. Organizational effectiveness.   2. Complex organizations.
3. Leadership.   4. Interorganizational relations.   I. Lorentz, Elizabeth.   II. Title.
HD58.9.S27   1998
    302.3'5—dc21   97-21221

FIRST EDITION
HB Printing   10 9 8 7 6 5 4 3 2 1

Contents

Contents

Preface

The authors have collaborated on two previous books. Despite this, our friendship and affection for each other have not diminished. That, we assume, is no small feat. Each of us has contributed to the other's intellectual and conceptual growth—an example of what in this book we call productive, asset enhancing resource exchange— and to whatever merits this book may have.

In our earlier writings, we said little about the applicability of our conceptions of resource exchange, coordination, and coordinators to the private and governmental sectors. Indeed, we regarded those sectors as so mired in the past and so imprisoned in the acceptance of bureaucratic ways of thinking and organizing that we saw no hope that what we had demonstrated and advocated would be understood, let alone accepted. But, to our surprise, some organizational theorists and company executives have begun to adopt (out of sheer necessity) an orientation similar to ours. We do not want to exaggerate the significance of these instances, i.e., what they herald for the future. Clearly, though, there are stirrings of change, and we had to note and discuss them. It was these stirrings that compelled us to take up a question we had previously discussed only briefly: What are the characteristics of a resource exchange, boundary crossing coordinator? Finally, we wanted in this book to spell out—to give compelling instances of—the difference between a preventive approach that rivets on pathology, on what is wrong with people and the organizations in which they work, and one that seeks to promote "health" by locating, exploiting, and building on people's assets and strengths. The former is the dominant, or "medical model," approach—which, of course, has its place; the latter is one that shifts the emphasis to the actual or potential assets of people, assets that the organization chart mentality cannot recognize and even punishes, wittingly and unwittingly.

Vice President Al Gore took up these themes in his "Reinventing Government" program. In terms of recognizing and capitalizing on people's assets and strengths, of the necessity of boundary crossings for the purposes of resource exchange, of how limited resources need not be as limited as they appear to be, of how "added value" accrues through resource exchange—in regard to these parts of his rationale, it is as if he had read our books, which, of course, he had not. But that is one of the reasons for writing this book: different people in different kinds of public and private organizations have felt compelled to take the obvious seriously. And the obvious is that conventional organizational thinking is wasteful, impoverishing, and self-defeating.

Although we consider what we say in this book to be applicable to the life and structure of all formal organizations as well as their potential interconnectedness with each other, our focus is a more modest one: the need for recognition of an essential though generally informal coordinating role. The potential practical implications of this role are considerable, and they fall largely outside the existing literature on coordination and collaboration.

That literature has two features. The more obvious is that a major source of organizational inefficiency is flawed coordination and collaboration, regardless of how one distinguishes between the two concepts. The second is that "repairing" inefficiency is an uphill battle in which success is by no means assured and for which evidence that the success has been sustained and institutionalized is not robust. That there have been notable successes cannot (and should not) be denied. The literature contains overwhelmingly more instances of successes than failures, if only because those whose efforts failed do not tend to write about their experiences. It is also the case that editors of journals tend to see no point in accepting accounts of failure.

Nonetheless, all this literature on coordination and collaboration—large in volume, theoretically and practically productive, and by no means irrelevant to our work—does not reflect what we think is distinctive about our focus. There are a host of studies available to review, each of which has a confirming element illustrative of some aspect of our rationale, but none of which addresses the mode of action our rationale dictates. We therefore spend relatively little time with the literature in this volume, turning instead primarily to our own direct experience. Our way of thinking emerged not from armchair musings but from various efforts over the years to implement and test our ideas.

This book proceeds without attempting to define *coordination* and *collaboration* or distinguish between them. Such definitions and distinctions bypass the conceptual rationale and style of action that are central to our approach, and we had no desire to coin a new term. The words are already used in the literature with various related but subtly differing meanings, and they serve well for our distinctive conceptual rationale and the process of implementing it.

This book also makes no attempt to deal with coordination in all of its aspects. Instead, as noted earlier, we concentrate on a role that does not now exist within or among formal organizations, a role that some people play in their neighborhoods, communities, and the informal networks of which they are part and in which they "naturally" serve the coordinating, resource exchange function. No one seems to select these people; others just gravitate to the role. They would be nonplussed if they were told they had selected themselves for a role. They do what they do and have no need to conceptualize what they do, and they certainly have no need to write about it.

But there is a great deal to be learned from these people: their characteristics, personal style, accomplishments. Is there a place for them in formal organizations? The fact is that there are such people in formal organizations—but they go unrecognized because the organizational ethos and structure pose insuperable obstacles both to their formal recognition and their proper use. Formal organizations tend to treat people as differentiated resources; workers are slotted and pigeonholed, and woe unto those who do not stay within the confines of their carefully crafted job descriptions.

Some organizational theorists have told us that although they wholeheartedly agree with the thrust of our rationale, the role we describe is too ambiguous, too messy, for an organization to tolerate and sustain. In the examples we present, the theorists are proved correct in regard to the appearance of messiness, except that they are quite wrong in that the fruits of that messiness more than compensate for its problems. As is so often true, logic here provides a systematic way of going wrong with complete confidence. It can also be a mammoth barrier to taking seriously a new idea embedded in a rationale different from the one the logic supports.

Obviously, we consider the term *messy* inappropriate and misleading. As best we could determine, the few individuals who used that term had difficulty conceiving of a coordinating role that at the same time was informal in style while having formal institutionalized support and recognition. The problem has not been that *aspects* of the role are not performed by anyone in formal organizations. That is not always the case (even though it is so in most formal organizations). The problem is that the significance and potentialities of the role are neither recognized nor supported, nor exploited. It is the purpose of this book to indicate the wastefulness of this situation and to describe and discuss a way of thinking about and dealing with it.

Plan of the Book

Experience has taught us that although our conceptual rationale brings ready assent, it tends to be an agreement in the abstract and not rooted in the assenters' concrete experience. Yet we did not want to overwhelm the reader with example after example of the "problem of coordination." Initially, we planned to draw on our long and extensive experience in the schools. It would be a relatively simple matter to organize a book largely around the schools' intractability to change and improvement and their relation to issues of coordination and collegiality. On the other hand, we decided that putting schools center stage would be reinforcing the myth that schools are unique organizations having little or no— certainly no major—commonalities with private-sector, governmental, or nonprofit organizations. But schools are not unique entities. They are different, but they do not require special theories or rationales, any more than the fact that oxygen and helium atoms are different means you need a special theory for each. It often seems that failure to recognize this point has prevented educational theorists and reformers from applying lessons learned from other types of organizations.

It is the bedrock of our thinking that issues of coordination and collegiality are of general significance in all organizations, specifically including the schools, and we are particularly interested— because of our long years of work in the field—in seeing this point taken seriously by educational theorists and reformers. We fear that our schools will remain what they are or get worse until the need for coordination gains recognition. To strike a balance between specific relevance to the schools and the general significance of the themes of this book, we have used the schools as a frame. The introduction and the epilogue address the concerns of the schools directly, while the body of the book speaks of them only in passing.

In the introduction, we discuss the charter schools that are being established across the country in an effort to develop new approaches to school reform. Charter schools reflect, among other things, a long overdue recognition of an educational system in which coordination of the parts is distinguished by its absence and in which the assets of the diverse members are not exploited. To use the vice president's apt phrase about government, it is a system that sustains a "culture of futility."

In the years since publication of our earlier books, with their pessimistic view of the future of collaboration and coordination in formal organizations, it has become clear that something akin to a paradigm shift is occurring. Chapter One discusses paradigm shifts in general and as applied to organizational life, using as illustrations Gore's Reinventing Government program and its great and successful predecessor, the Constitutional Convention of 1787. The defining documents for the vice president's program explicitly address sources of the heretofore intractable problem of coordination. The three documents—which, apparently, few people have read or will read—deserve the closest scrutiny because of what they say about redefinition of people as resources, resource exchange, and boundary crossing. However, even though we praise these reports from the standpoint of rationale and diagnosis, we are critical of their lack of specificity about the roles and processes that implementation requires. Who will play coordinating roles? How will they be selected and on what basis? What will be required to sustain the process? Is there a place for a person in a coordinating role who has no power but who, possessing the characteristics we described, starts the network process and creates forums that make resource exchange and boundary crossing possible and productive? Where do you start, and by what criteria? How do you avoid confirming the maxim that the more things change the more they remain the same?

Chapters Two through Six explore the general significance of five key themes essential to the application of the new paradigm: the way we ordinarily define people as resources, the obstacles to redefinition of resources, the role of networks for maximizing the application of resources, the special role and characteristics of the network coordinator, and the way resource exchange energizes and reinforces collegiality and a sense of community.

Chapter Two addresses the question of defining resources, pointing out that the definition itself can effectively reduce the resources available to an organization. A job description delineates what a person is expected to do; it implies that he or she does not possess knowledge and talents the organization could exploit. In practice, and far more often than not, the job description means "You do what you were hired to do, and do not cross boundaries."

In Chapter Three, we take up a subtle but comprehensive obstacle to applying the new paradigm: the imagery of mechanics built into the organization chart, with its implicit assumption that if all parts are assembled in appropriate ways there will be a desirable outcome. We do not recommend abandoning organization charts, but we point out the pitfalls of confusing the intentions of a chart with their realization.

Chapter Four briefly summarizes our earlier experience and then takes up the fascinating and bedeviling question: What is the combination of characteristics a coordinator should have? We begin the answer by returning to Mrs. Dewar, who held center stage in our earlier books. In the years following the publication of those books (Sarason & Lorentz, 1979/1989a, Sarason & others, 1977/1989b), it has become known that "Mrs. Dewar" is in fact Elizabeth M. Lorentz herself; but we have retained the name here for continuity's sake. Although she is doubtless not unique, we know of no one like her who has been described in detail elsewhere. The role she played does not exist in formal organizations. We have reason to believe that the others remain unknown precisely because their role is an informal one, and it never enters their minds that what they do should be written up. What they are and do are not of much interest to social science researchers, at least not to a degree that would lead theorists and researchers to observe and describe these people with the detail they deserve.

Building on the fourth chapter, Chapter Five has two purposes. It describes the characteristics of the coordinator under four headings: knowing the territory; scanning, fluidity, imaginativeness; perceiving assets and building on strengths; and power, influence, and selflessness. We strive to put flesh on the bones of those abstractions by describing people who, we came to learn, have some of those characteristics. The second purpose is to begin to describe how one selects people who appear to have the proper *combination* of characteristics. We italicize combination to emphasize that any one of the characteristics can be found in many individuals; it is their combination that is crucial for the resource exchange, boundary crossing role.

Chapter Six extends the discussion of the paradigm shift to the private sector, describing insights that have begun to appear among a small number of organizational theorists and consultants, as well as among some business executives whose companies were on the road to failure. It provides examples of how resource exchange and collaboration bring new life to organizations in both the private and the public sectors, extending their reach and their ability to influence their worlds. We note that however heartening these changes are, the kind of description of process that makes evaluation, or even approximate replication, possible is lacking. But we no longer doubt that the challenge to outmoded assumptions of how organizations should be structured and run has appeared on the horizon.

The epilogue returns to the authors' ongoing concern with the public schools. Schools as they are cannot be comprehended unless one understands how their organizational features—undergirded by the organization chart mentality—were influenced by the private-sector mode of organization that developed in the early years of the twentieth century, an influence continuing today. Our schools are organizationally the direct descendants of schools developed to tame and socialize children of the waves of immigrants in the nineteenth century and the early decades of the twentieth, and their organizational features were mightily influenced by the rationale for the factories of those times. The new organizational paradigm we describe in this book has hardly begun to apply in the educational arena, but as far back as a century ago there were a few critics of the public schools who not only saw what a disaster it would be if schools continued to be organized and run like the factories of those times, but who also presented a rationale surprisingly similar to what organizational theorists and practitioners began to advocate in the post–World War II era. Meanwhile, it is well worth considering the schools in detail. If they remain as inadequate as they are, the consequences will be increasingly destabilizing for the entire society. That is not a pleasant prospect. As long as we view schools as a unique type of organization—not only different but unique—we blind ourselves to the problems they share with the private sector and our public agencies, *and for the same reasons.*

Acknowledgments

There may be readers interested in the creation, activities, and accomplishments of our resource exchange network (the Northern Westchester Resource Network), discussed in Chapter Four. In addition to our two earlier books, we suggest that such readers consult Virginia Thompson's doctoral dissertation, completed in 1985 at Teachers College, Columbia University (Thompson, 1985). Her aim was not only to describe how members of that network viewed its purposes and activities but also to come to conclusions about how well the network fulfilled its stated purposes. That her conclusions warmed our hearts goes without saying. But it is not a study uncritical of that network. She raises some important issues, which we endeavor in this book to discuss.

We are to no end delighted to acknowledge that somehow or other Lisa Pagliaro, as usual, managed to type the final draft without a personal breakdown. Sarason writes in longhand, which is problem enough, and Lorentz's handwriting also borders on the indecipherable—nevertheless, unflappable Lisa stayed the course. In the usual organization chart, Lisa would be in a box labeled typist or secretary. That would be as clear an example of a fact obscuring the truth, of assets and strengths ignored, as we know.

August 1997   Seymour B. Sarason
                                                                 Stratford, Connecticut

                                                                 Elizabeth M. Lorentz
                                                                 Armonk, New York

The Authors

Seymour B. Sarason is professor of psychology emeritus in the Department of Psychology and at the Institute for Social and Policy Studies at Yale University. He founded, in 1962, and directed until 1970, the Yale Psycho-Educational Clinic, one of the first research and training sites in community psychology. He received his Ph.D. degree (1942) from Clark University and holds honorary doctorates from Syracuse University, Queens College, Rhode Island College, and Lewis and Clark College. He has received an award for distinguished contributions to the public interest and several awards from the divisions of clinical and community psychology of the American Psychological Association, as well as two awards from the American Association on Mental Deficiency.

Sarason is the author of numerous books and articles. His more recent books include *The Making of an American Psychologist: An Autobiography* (1980); *The Predictable Failure of Educational Reform: Can We Change Course Before It's Too Late?* (1990); *The Challenge of Art to Psychology* (1990); *You Are Thinking of Teaching? Opportunities, Problems, Realities* (1993); *The Case for Change: Rethinking the Preparation of Educators* (1993); *Letters to a Serious Education President* (1993); *Psychoanalysis, General Custer, and the Verdicts of History and Other Essays on Psychology in the Social Scene* (1994); *Parental Involvement and the Political Principle: Why the Existing Governance Structure of Schools Should Be Abolished* (1995); and *Barometers of Change: Individual, Educational, and Social Transformation* (1996).

Elizabeth M. Lorentz supervises new coordinators of resource exchange networks in the New York metropolitan area. She also brings network concepts to bear on the organizations on whose advisory boards she serves, including the Institute for Responsive Education, the Bank Street College of Education, the College for Human Services, the Rene Dubos Forum, and the Public Education Association.

Lorentz gained a generalist background by doing research and reports for directors of government agencies and magazine editors who wanted briefing on developments in various fields of human service. In the process, she became convinced that services by specialist professions and agencies would only be integrated if the lay citizen got involved.

Crossing Boundaries

Introduction: Charters, Curricula, and a History of Failure

The future of this society will in large measure be decided by what happens in the effort to change and improve schooling. But that effort will not succeed as long as schools are regarded as unique organizations for whom what has been learned about other types of organizations is considered irrelevant. As this book demonstrates, the concepts of coordination and collegiality are key to all organizations in this last decade of the twentieth century, and to none more than the schools, which need them most and seem to be lagging furthest behind in the new development.

Readers of this book will all doubtless have heard about charter schools: those explicit, deliberate attempts on the part of state leadership to create schools relatively independent of existing school systems. The charter school movement rests on the diagnosis that existing school systems are inimical and intractable to achieving improved educational outcomes. Almost every state has passed enabling legislation (in 1996, the Connecticut legislature created twenty-four such charter schools). It is hard to exaggerate the importance of the charter school; it is the first attempt to do something *radical* about school reform. It rests on one assumption and one hope. The assumption—never verbalized but always left implicit—is that schools and school systems are or may be unrescuable. The hope is, of course, that the charter school will provide instructive data to those responsible for educational policy. Since charter schools will receive the same per capita support as traditional schools (or slightly more), then if they are successful (more productive of desirable outcomes) the implications are, to say the least, enormous.

From our perspective, several questions have to be asked. In each state, each of the charter schools is for all practical purposes on its own, i.e., it will determine how it will use its fiscal and human resources to achieve the purposes stated in applying for special status. So the first question is: What will be the relationship among these schools embarked on uncharted seas? We are familiar with the legislation and implementation in several states. The fact is that nothing is said or being done about how these schools can be of help to each other. As Sarason pointed out a quarter of a century ago (1972), the creation of a new setting brings in its wake certain predictable problems: the creators almost always underestimate the complexity of creating a new setting; it is the opposite of an easy act, and they are not prepared to deal with it. In addition, if anything is predictable about creating a new setting, it is that unpredictable problems will be encountered, e.g., something happens to the leader, the inadequacies of this or that staff member become manifest, "outside" opposition or criticisms appear.

The new, encapsulated charter schools will experience similar kinds of problems, however different their written application, mode of organization, and pedagogy may be. It is also predictable that some of these schools will cope more effectively with these issues than others. It is inconceivable that these schools have nothing to give or take from each other, and that the giving and taking will assume many forms. From our perspective, this is not only a glimpse of the obvious but the beginning step in what we regard as a crucial goal: how to define and apply existing resources so that they are mutually and productively enlarged and *exchanged*. We italicize the word *exchanged* because it implies a degree of mutual understanding and knowledge that makes for a discernible increase in the productive use of existing resources. Someone said that money is a necessary means of exchange among strangers. But when money is absent or realistically not in the picture, one is still left with the power of an informal connectedness that makes for mutual understanding and a willing exchange of resources. Unfortunately, such connectedness does not exist among charter schools.

Each has the assets and deficits of a rampant, rugged individualism.

What would we have recommended? We would have recommended that money be provided to create a position whose incumbent would have several responsibilities as well as restrictions:

- The individual would need to become knowledgeable about each school in a given area: its different personnel and stakeholders, its forums for discussion and decision making. The overriding responsibility of the person is to know the schools well enough, and to have established his or her interpersonal credentials well enough, to be able to determine when people in different schools need each other and bring them together in ways that are practical and mutually productive.
- It would be made clear that the person has no power to require anyone in any school to do anything. He or she will not report to any higher authority.
- The stated responsibility of the person is to suggest how the resources, ideas, and problems of school A might be helpful to school B, etc. If the suggestion is accepted, the individual arranges a meeting between the relevant personnel in the schools. The individual moderates the meeting but doesn't own or control it.
- Any school that does not wish to use the services of the person does not need to do so.

In this book we label this role *network coordinator*, and we describe and discuss it in detail in later chapters. Far more important than a job label is what the person does and why. To our knowledge, no such full-time role exists in or among formal organizations. Our network experience, which is considerable, confirms that *requiring* coordination or collaboration is an exercise in futility. So are exhortations that appeal to the institutional obligations individuals should feel. Unless people see it as in their immediate self-interest voluntarily and safely to consider and explore bridge building, whatever you mean by coordination and collaboration will not likely occur and survive. In principle, that is precisely the rationale for charter schools: to give people the opportunity to practice in ways that make personal sense to them, ways that do not require them to conform to the dictates of the system at the expense of what they find personally and conceptually salient. But the current charter school programs reinforce this independence with organizational walls, providing no opportunity for participants to voluntarily extend their practice to include mutual information sharing and resource exchange. It would magnify the power of each charter school manyfold to have a reliable but noncoercive bridge to its fellows, that is, a network coordinator as we define the position here.

What are the characteristics of a network coordinator? As later chapters will indicate, it is a crucial question because the role requires a particular way of viewing people as multifaceted resources (regardless of job titles), a capacity to scan settings in terms of resources and new possibilities for interconnecting and exploiting them, and a willingness to be in a role with no formal power but with the potential to serve as a catalyst and enable others to see themselves and others in new and productive ways. Selecting people for such a role is not easy, and neither is performing in the role.

Comparing Industry and the Public Schools

How is any complex task—whether the assembly of an automobile or computer or the education of a child—accomplished? It would take a book of some size to answer that question. But one thing we know: it is a process consisting of steps, each one of which has to be coordinated with those that have gone before, and coordinated in a way that is smooth, is efficient, and avoids costly malfunctions. It may appear to be a "mindless" process until something goes wrong, at which point an effort is made to determine where and why the coordination has failed. Is it faulty material? A systematic human error? An inadequate conception of how steps in the process should be coordinated? Is it that those involved in one step of the process have no knowledge of or interest in the previous or subsequent steps, i.e., they have no picture of how and why they are related to other steps?

If any lesson has been learned from Japan's startling industrial success, it is that emphasis is placed on issues of coordination *within and among* steps of production, an emphasis requiring a high degree of collegiality irrespective of status. The quality of the final product is not determined at the end of production but at every step of the way so as to drastically lessen the high cost of corrections in a product already assembled. That means that at every step everyone's knowledge, perceptions, and opinions are sought. Quality of product depends in large part on the quality of information elicited in the process of production. To American executives and managers imprisoned in a narrow assembly-line way of thinking, the Japanese approach seemed costly in time and, therefore, in the size of the bottom line. They learned the hard way: the superior quality of Japanese autos slowly and steadily resulted in a very significant increase in market share. Japanese workers and managers may have spent more time "talking," but they produced a product superior to that of their American counterparts.

Now let us look at the American production process of education from the standpoint of coordination of its different steps. For many children, the first step antedates entry into the public school; some children have been in a nursery school or a Head Start program. The second step is entry into a kindergarten—which to most teachers in the elementary school is not "real" school but preparation for it. The third step is entry into the first grade. Depending on local educational philosophy and fiscal exigencies, the elementary school may have as few as three and as many as five discrete steps. Then there are the middle school steps, followed by those in the high school. In brief, the child experiences many steps, and the underlying assumption is that when a child leaves his or her teacher in step A, the child is prepared for what the new teacher will do in step B. But what does the expectation imply? At the very least, it implies that the teacher in step B knows what knowledge, skills, and attitudes the teacher in step A has inculcated and fostered. It also implies that the two teachers have not worked in isolation from each other but rather have discussed and worked through how their efforts and goals can be coordinated in ways productive not for children in the abstract but for the real students going from teacher A to teacher B. We assume that teacher A has learned a great deal about each student that teacher B will get, e.g., his or her learning style and habits, motivation, vulnerabilities, personality, sociability, and more. Is that knowledge irrelevant to teacher B's purposes? Is it of such minor importance as not to justify the time required for the knowledge to be mined and discussed? Is it sufficient for teacher A only to certify that the children are "ready" for the next step? In fact, it is the exception and not the rule for teachers A and B to have developed the degree of collegiality that is the basis of productive coordination. The steps in the educational process are coordinated in theory and given expression in what is termed the curriculum. However, descriptions of the curriculum tend to suggest a degree of coordination and collegiality that is no more a reflection of reality than are the organization charts of most private-sector organizations.

One of the more blatant examples of what we are criticizing occurs when students go from the elementary to the middle school. Not only is the middle school significantly larger in size and population than the elementary school but it is organized along departmental lines. Whereas in the elementary school the student has spent most of the day with one teacher, in the middle school he or she may have five different teachers, each of whom may be in a different department. What do these teachers know about students catapulted into a far more organizationally differentiated school than the one to which they have been accustomed? The answer is: next to nothing. It is no secret that relations between the elementary and the middle school are like those between two foreign countries. Records accompany the students—they are on file in the principal's office—but few teachers if any read them unless the behavior or academic performance of a student is problematic, and even then the records are more often than not uninformative. In describing the relations between the elementary and middle school, the words *coordination* and *collegiality* do not come to mind. Here again, the underlying assumption seems to be that the middle school needs to know only that students have been certified to be ready for the middle school experience. Again it is no secret in the educational community that in the middle school an increase in behavior and academic problems becomes very noticeable and student disengagement and boredom are hard to ignore.

We are not asserting that these manifestations are explained only by an absence of coordination and collegiality; this would be an oversimple explanation. But we do assert that the absence of coordination and collegiality between the elementary and middle school, *and* a similar absence *within* the middle school, have to be part of the explanation. The same holds in spades for the relation between the middle and the high school, *and* within the much larger high school.

In the industrial sector, production steps are geared to put out uniform products for which there is reason to believe there have been satisfied customers in the past and there will be more in the future. In the production steps of our educational system, it is known from the very first step that at the final step there will be no "uniform product" because each child is truly unique in the way in which such factors as temperament, ability, motivation, curiosity, personal style, etc., are patterned. Those factors are not independent of social-cultural-familial variables. Such uniqueness is implied in the often heard statement that "the aim of schooling is to help each child realize his or her full potential." This is to say, at the end of the final step of schooling students will vary considerably in performance (and much more), but it is the purpose of schooling to get the best out of each student by knowing and capitalizing on the student's individuality. However, the rhetoric is belied by the reality that the educational production line is not geared to take individuality seriously. The reasons are many; we have chosen here to illustrate the issue by focusing on what passes for coordination and collegiality because they are processes and relationships through which "knowing" a child becomes a possibility. Where there is incoordination and an absence of collegiality— and where both become more glaring as the student traverses the many steps—the rhetoric of individuality should be recognized for what it is: empty.

A group of CEOs from private industry recently got together in a "summit conference" on education. In the conference report (*A 1996 National Education Summit Policy Statement*, 1996), the words *standards*, *high expectations*, and *technology* appear with high frequency. This conveys a strong impression that the conference participants blame school personnel for the present plight of our schools. That is to say, the report seems to assert that school personnel have accepted low standards of academic performance, they expect too little from their students and they get little, and they have not provided students the incentives or conditions to meet high and necessary standards of performance. Coming as it does from executives of large companies, the diagnosis is strange indeed. In their own bailiwicks and from their personal experience, they know—they truly know—that when a complicated organization is steadily failing, the explanation is far less in the failings of individuals than in *a system and organizational culture* that is self-defeatingly coordinated, in which divisiveness within and between parts is the rule and not the exception, and in which pressures for change are effectively withstood.

The report states and restates how essential it is to obtain agreement about goals, needed skills, and "authentic and accurate systems to tell us how well school and students are doing." This theme is preceded by "We recognize that better use of technology, improved curriculum, better trained educators, and other changes in the organization and management of schools are necessary to facilitate improved school performance." No one, of course, disputes the importance of agreement on goals. But as the history of educational reform well documents, the level of agreement has foundered on the inability to get agreement about what constitutes "changes in the organization and management of schools." Schools have a distinctive culture, a culture in which what is a resource, who is a resource, and how resources are to be coordinated and employed have a long history (Sarason, 1990, 1996). It is a culture in which community and collegiality are notably absent or weak, setting drastic limits to effective coordination of resources. That is the point: the statement calls for a degree and quality of coordination, a redefinition of resources, that is not obtainable by a verbal agreement about academic goals, however sincere the verbal agreement may be. Between verbal agreement and actions consistent with it is a minefield of obstacles that has made for several generations of burned-out reformers who did not heed the caveat of the anthropologist: when you seek to intervene in a "foreign" culture, your first task is to understand the culture in its own terms. For example, the CEOs' report talks about schools as if a school were *not* part of a complicated, hierarchically organized *system* the parts of which have conflicting interests, a turf-protective stance, and a zero-sum orientation in regard to resource allocation. On an organization chart, these parts appear coordinated, whereas in "real life" they are not; on this, few teachers and other educators would disagree. Nor would all but a few contest the assertion that collegiality and sense of common purpose are rare in a single school, let alone a school system. The same can be said about the relationship between schools and school systems on the one hand, and preparatory programs in universities on the other hand. Both types of institutions have different cultures, traditions, organizational features, and vested interests. Each needs the other, each has resources that should be coordinated in a mutually satisfactory way, and each employs rhetoric about satisfaction with their interactions, but the fact is that the rhetoric, far more often than not, covers up a reservoir of suspicion, hostility, wariness, and dissatisfaction.

The CEOs' prescription for school change does not address the relationship between the inadequacies of our public schools and the nature of the system in which those schools are embedded. It is far beyond the purposes of this book to discuss the nature of the system and how it guarantees that the more things change the more they will remain the same (Sarason, 1996). Our purpose here is both more limited and more general: we seek to demonstrate that in trying to understand failing, troubled organizations, a productive beginning point is to examine issues surrounding coordination and collegiality. We hope to demonstrate that when organizations change in positive and productive ways, issues of coordination and collegiality take on a new and more hopeful cast, and problems that previously appeared insoluble reshape themselves in more tractable terms—if not turn into outright advantages.

Stepping and Stumbling

The CEOs' report is far from the first in the field, and not the only one to ignore its predecessors. In the sizzling sixties, the public schools became a focus of controversy as their inadequacies, rigidities, and resistance to change became apparent. People criticized the schools not only for their internal structure, system, and culture but also for their inadequate relationships with the community at large and community agencies. What began was the formal creation of task forces at the federal, state, and local levels to alter both the internal features of schools and school systems and their relationships to other community agencies and resources as well. Of course, a prominent feature of these task forces' charge was a new coordination of services and resources.

At one point, the authors of this book took on the awesome task of trying to read and digest the reports each state was legislatively required to prepare, as well as a sample of the reports of local groups. We tried to read the many reports emanating from the federal department of education, culminating in the heralded, promoted, Reagan-appointed commission report *A Nation at Risk* (National Council on Excellence in Education, 1983).

If our task was awesome, it was also impossible psychologically and timewise. But we pursued it long enough to conclude with confidence that each report stands alone. None of them contains the faintest hint that similar reports with similar purposes (albeit under different auspices) had been written over and over again, with little or no productive consequences.

History does not tell us what we should do about the specific problems we are confronting today; history does not provide us with a blueprint for action. But history can tell us what we should be thinking about, what errors of omission and commission have been made, what potholes have remained uncovered, and why these past efforts have been so unproductive. So, for example, in everything we have read today and whatever we have learned from talking to relevant staff about "reinventing" government, we have discerned no interest whatsoever in the question of why the scores of similar efforts in the past (starting, say, with the Hoover Commission) have been so barren of results. We are aware that those past efforts did not deal exclusively with coordination—but there was never any doubt that issues of coordination were or would be crucial. The imagery of the mechanical assembly of parts suffuses these reports, as it does the reports of today and the organization chart mentality of public and private business that we discuss in detail in Chapter Three. These were well-intentioned, necessary efforts. They did not, however, confront the realities of the customary relationships of parts, agencies, departments, and the like, and those relationships rose up and swallowed almost every vestige of improvement the reports' sponsors hoped to see. History unexamined does repeat itself over and over, but there is always an opportunity to make a break and begin to build something new.

Chapter One

An Emerging Paradigm Shift

We are used to hearing about paradigm shifts: replacing one customary way of thinking with a new one that is more explanatory of important problems than the old one, and more productive of usable knowledge (theoretical or practical). Newtonian physics supplanted the Copernican paradigm, and Einsteinian physics supplanted the Newtonian paradigm. Paradigm shifts do not necessarily mean that what has been replaced was completely wrong. What they do mean is that certain specified problems were wrongly or incompletely explained and the new explanation is a far better one.

In the case of organizational theory and practice, the problem that has proved most intractable has been coordination of people and resources. Proposed explanations have directed attention to one or another aspect of human behavior, such as managerial style, adversarialism, complacency, rigidity, and other human frailties. What was behind these explanations was the paradigm of the organization as consisting of bounded parts within each of which were people possessing certain skills not possessed by those in other parts. More than that, people in one part were not *expected* to possess knowledge or ideas of practical value to people in other parts. Coordination was the responsibility of department heads who, if they were good women or men (that is, if they were appropriately motivated), would ensure coordination.

Today we know that explanations based on that paradigm are inadequate philosophically, theoretically, and practically. Vice President Gore's reports on reinventing government—discussed in some detail later in this chapter—are refreshing precisely because they reject that paradigm and cite the experience and writings of others as justification for the rejection. And they come up with a new, boundary crossing rationale or paradigm. So far so good. But the justification for a new paradigm is not in the newness of the theory; rather, it is in the demonstration in practice that an intractable problem can be overcome. That is, the new theory must have been used in the development of new methods, and those methods must have been employed and shown to produce the desired results.

We fully agree with the new rationale.[1] But the reinventing-government documents contain little or no indication that these new methods are being devised. There is much about crossing boundaries, forming teams, and liberating the creativity of people. Those are goals, not methods, strategies, or tactics. So it is not surprising that the entire report contains no hint that new roles may need to be created, roles that do not now exist, roles that cannot even be imagined because the vice president and his staff are still prisoners of the old paradigm—as indeed they must be. Embracing a new paradigm does not mean that the old one is no longer in your psychological bloodstream; anyone who has experienced a paradigm shift knows that. It may well be that no one can fully plumb the implications of a paradigm shift. For this to happen requires a variety of people each of whom embraces the paradigm in idiosyncratic ways, thereby revealing implications none of them can see alone.

Today we are used to hearing that we have entered the era of the "global village," where ultimately everyone will be connected with everyone else, where what happens in one place will be known to and have an impact upon what happens everyplace else. There is a difference between being connected and being coordinated, however. One can regard the words *global village* as an oxymoron if by village you intend the imagery of people very much known to each other and aware of their dependence on each other, and of a place where the informal is at least as important as the formal (if not more important), where bartering and resource exchange are frequent, and where no one has to be taught the significance of interdependence. That may be an idealized picture, but it is one we cherish because it is so different from what we experience in our social and working lives as well as in the happenings around the rest of the world. It is not fortuitous that almost all those who seriously talk about the global village come from the scientific-technologic arenas, where the imagery of computers, faxes, and communication satellites abounds. (It is not unlike the imagery that gives rise to complicated organization charts.) Although the world can be so connected, this does not mean that it is being coordinated so as to make the use of resources, human and material, more productive of mutually enhancing growth. Just as one hopes that there is a paradigm shift in regard to organizational structure, dynamics, and purposes, one hopes that the same paradigm shift will change and inform the imagery of the global village.

From Theory to Practice

Applying the new paradigm is no simple matter. We know far less than we need to about how organizations are created, how they are changed, and the outcomes of such efforts—despite the fact that you can fill a rather large library with books and journals dealing with those questions. This is because descriptions of cases tend to be woefully inadequate or incomplete, not engendering in a reader a sense of security that he or she knows what went on. We may be given enough to be secure about the rationale employed and even, in a more general way, the criteria by which success or failure was to be judged. But in between explication of rationale and narration of outcomes is a poorly lit black box or cloud chamber. This situation is unsurprising, as filling in the black box is very time consuming, requires more than one person, and can be expensive.

Let us put it in this way: what is called for is the difference between a superficial and a comprehensive biography. A biography is a narrative of a life, and the biographer knows ahead of time that the finished account will still contain mystery and unanswered questions; but the best biographers strive to be as comprehensive as possible, to convey a sense of wholeness to the reader. So when we are told that a biography was authorized, we assume it is very likely we are not going to be told everything that is known or can be known about the person. But as any self-respecting biographer will attest, even when the biography is not authorized the biographer inevitably has a point of view that influences the material he or she selects and how "facts" are interpreted. That is why for any historically important person there usually is more than one biography. The important point is that the serious biographer seeks to be comprehensive, to get the reader to conclude that he or she knows the historic figure. In regard to the concerns of this book, we hardly have such descriptions of organizational structure, processes, dynamics, and social relationships.

For example, Lipnack and Stamps authored two books, *The Team Net Factor* (1993) and *The Age of the Network* (1994). These books are very intriguing to us because they contain examples from here and abroad of private-sector organizations employing a rationale similar to ours. Alone, each of the private-sector organizations the books describe either would have failed or stagnated or simply would have been unable creatively to capitalize on the assets they had. But those books neglect several interesting questions: In any one instance (say, the flexible manufacturing networks in northern Italy), who were the initiating actors? How did they begin and with whom? What problems were encountered? How were problems overcome? What means were employed or forums created where the possibilities of coordination could be discussed and strategies outlined? What kept the process going, and what were the characteristics of those who were most crucial—and at what points? Was any one instance a screaming success (which is unlikely), and what factors limited the degree of success? We, at least, found the descriptions wanting, too sketchy, too incomplete, to allow us to answer these questions and conclude that we know how the process began and was sustained. Coordination is not a process that, like

Topsy, just happens and grows. Partisans as we are for the rationale Lipnack and Stamps too briefly spell out, we believe that the outcomes they glowingly describe are not surprising. But this is an act of faith on our part. For our present purposes, their books are unrevealing as to how productive resource exchange and coordination came about and the status and style of those who were in coordinating roles. Anyone seeking to use their rationale; or to replicate what they say happened; or to evaluate the relationships between rationale, process, and outcomes cannot use the contents of their books as a dependable guide. Indubitably, however, Lipnack and Stamps have given currency to ideas that seem to be taking hold in private-sector organizations. Put another way, their imagery of coordination comes close to being the polar opposite of the conventional imagery of insular organizations and subgroups. For that they deserve a high grade. For description, the grade is much lower.

The absence of description plagues all aspects of work in this area. For example, probably more than any other state Oregon has taken Gore's Reinventing Government seriously. As best as we can determine from materials made available to us and from telephone conversations, the conception of networks and coordinators sounds encouraging. Still, we do not have anything resembling a description that even begins to answer the questions we have just asked. What is encouraging is that we have recently learned that Oregon has hired a "journalist" (their term) to describe what is going on. Unfortunately, the federal government has not seen fit to do anything similar. Given the frailties of institutional memory, we will end up with anecdotes, opinions, and uninstructive generalizations, from none of which can we expect to learn anything.

We are reminded here of the Job Corps, started in the sixties as part of the war on poverty. Senator Daniel Moynihan had the good sense to realize at the time that the objectives of the Job Corps were very similar to those of the CCC (Civilian Conservation Corps) created during the Great Depression thirty years earlier. What did we learn about the CCC? What had been the problems? Since it was regarded as a success, how was that explained? Senator

Moynihan started on the quest of locating reports relevant to these questions. He gave up. No such reports existed.

Reinventing Government in the Twentieth Century

It is useful to consider Vice President Gore's project, Reinventing Government, in some detail: its rationale, scope, diagnoses, and strategies, and its implications for the kind of description we would need to assess its accomplishments and failures. The groundwork for the project is given in three documents we consider models of candor and conceptualization. In regard to previous analyses of governmental inefficiencies reflective of the worst features of the bureaucratic mentality, these documents are refreshing in startling ways. The reader will be well served to read *From Red Tape to Results: Creating a Government That Works Better and Costs Less* and two similarly titled reports, subtitled *Transforming Organizational Structures* and *Strengthening the Partnership in Intergovernmental Service Delivery*, all published in 1993.

Given our purposes, we shall limit ourselves to what these reports say about coordination. This is not much of a limitation because coordination as a problem is frequently described, and where it is not it is implicitly in the picture. Let us start with what the report calls "The Root Problem."

> Is government inherently incompetent? Absolutely not. Are federal agencies filled with incompetent people? No. The problem is much deeper: Washington is filled with organizations designed for an environment that no longer exists—bureaucracies so big and wasteful they can no longer serve the American people. . . .
>
> In Washington's highly politicized world, the greatest risk is not that a program will perform poorly, but that a scandal will erupt. Scandals are front-page news, while routine failure is ignored. Hence control system after control system is piled up to minimize the risk of scandal. The budget system, the personnel rules, the procurement process, the inspectors general—all are designed to

prevent the tiniest misstep. We assume that we can't trust employees to make decisions, so we spell out in precise detail how they must do virtually everything, then audit them to ensure that they have obeyed every rule. The slightest deviation prompts new regulations and even more audits. . . . Federal employees quickly learn that common sense is risky—and creativity is downright dangerous. They learn that the goal is not to produce results, please customers, or save taxpayers' money, but to avoid mistakes. Those who dare to innovate do so quietly [1993a, pp. 3–5].

Here is a recommendation that recurs in all three reports: "Create partnerships within and between agencies and encourage crossing internal and external boundaries to integrate service delivery and policy development. The government should operate much like a 'boundaryless company,' where the primary loyalty of employees is serving citizen needs and where cross-agency work is commonplace. All relevant contributors and stakeholders should be included in planning and decision making to ensure that approaches to getting the work done are both effective and efficient" (1993a, p. 6).

Unlike previous reports, the reinventing-government documents mince no words in stating that the problem is a climate of fear and futility in which engaging in creative thinking and "crossing boundaries" confirms the adage that no good deed goes unpunished. But as the reports eloquently say in many of their pages, what is called the root problem is a direct consequence of the narrowest, self-defeating conception of the capabilities of people, a conception that essentially says that a person's contribution to the workplace will be worthy to the extent that he or she is told clearly and in detail precisely what to do, and by implication what not to do. (This is a good summary of the endemic social problem of the narrow definition of human resources, to which we return in Chapter Two.) The problem is less a distrust of people's judgment and more a fear of the unpredictable, of the inefficiencies that the boxes, arrows, and lines of the organization chart are supposed to prevent. We would emphasize that the usual job description conveys two messages: what a person will and should do, and what is off limits for that person. In any event, these reports are noteworthy for their damning criticisms of the kind of thinking discussed in Chapter Three, in which organization charts confuse intent with reality and the rationality reflected in chart making with efficiency in outcomes: a rationality that gives substance to the conclusion that logic is the systematic way of going wrong with complete confidence.

The reports go on at some length to recommend coordination and boundary crossing among agencies in terms that fit well with the premise of this book. However, its authors also note: "The Treasury, Postal Service, and General Appropriations Act of 1993 makes funding of interagency entities very difficult. Sometimes referred to as the 'anti-pass the hat' provision, it states that '*no part of any appropriation contained in this or any other Act shall be available for interagency financing of boards, commissions, councils, committees, or similar groups . . . which do not have a prior and specific statutory approval to receive financial support from more than one agency or instrumentality*'" (1993a, p. 17). In other words: feather your own nest, stay in your own bailiwick, and any thoughts you may have of engaging in "foreign affairs" had better remain in the realm of thought.

That provision reminds us of the story about an army colonel responsible for keeping a collection of records going back to the Civil War. He wrote a memo to his commanding officer saying that housing and protecting these ancient records was very expensive and truly unjustifiable. The commanding officer agreed but said he would have to pass the memo to higher authorities, and it finally got to the pertinent general. Back came the memo with the stamp of approval and an appended note saying: "Splendid idea. Just make sure to make carbons of what you destroy." The story is undoubtedly apocryphal—but the three reinventing-government reports contain instances no more comprehensible, and less funny.

Gore's efforts have given us a very clear, sophisticated, and compelling organizational diagnosis and rationale. In regard to issues only indirectly related to coordination, these reports tend to be incisive and concrete. However, in regard to coordination and boundary crossing, they are explicit only about one thing: coordination and boundary crossing will not be achieved by directive and fiat because those means will fuel the fires of resistance and resentment, i.e., they will be seen as but another top-down directive insensitive to an organizational climate of "fear and futility." Perhaps the most singular feature of these reports is the recognition that to criticize those who are objects of change is to blame the victim and ignore the fact that they are what they are and they think the way they think because of the ways they have been socialized, so to speak, into their organizational cultures.

So where do you start? Why here and not there? Who are *you*, the instigator of change? The last question implies but does not much clarify the obvious: in this context, *you* need to be someone with a grasp of the problem, commitment to its solution, and the status to get the ball rolling. The question can get you quickly on the road to infinite regression. Imagine that you are the vice president, and you have to decide where to start reinventing government and with whom. You have many responsibilities, and the time you can allot to the project is limited. Do you start with the Department of the Interior? Treasury? HUD? Agriculture? Where you start depends on how well you yourself possess one of the basic characteristics of a coordinator (a concept discussed in Chapter Five), the ability to answer the questions: How well do you know the territory? Who in your network is most likely to be receptive to your ideas? By *receptive* we mean someone whose self-interests are compatible with your ideas to the point where he or she would be willing to carry the ball in ways consistent with the spirit of those ideas. There is a difference between getting agreement in the abstract and getting agreement from someone whose self-interests make your position attractive and who accepts it willingly as a spur to action. But say the secretary of agriculture is no less busy than you (perhaps busier), with more things to do than he has time for. He has staff who themselves have staffs, and on and on down the hierarchy. What is required is that the secretary know the territory and select a person on precisely the same basis as your decision to select the secretary. Each step of the way is a step toward giving currency to ideas and ways of implementing them; we have found that this kind of currency can have the effect of "flushing out" individuals who want to be participants.

What one has to be alert to—what one seeks to avoid—is illustrated in a game teachers employ in the classroom. The teacher lines up the students and whispers a short message to a student who then has to whisper it to the next in line, and the whispering of messages goes on until the last student says the message aloud. Sometimes the "final" message bears resemblance to the original, but more frequently it does not. In the classroom, the message is short and simple. But the message Vice President Gore is conveying in the new paradigms of reinvented government is a complicated rationale, the implications and obligations of which are no simple matter. In addition, the process is not only a matter of selecting people who know the territory but also people who, you have reason to believe, possess other key characteristics of coordinators and boundary crossers. And let us not forget: we are describing a process in a system where power is rarely, if ever, *not* a factor in relationships. What you want people to consider as a suggestion, as a possibility, as something to mull over, can too easily be interpreted as a directive the recipients had better act on despite reservations or unexpressed disagreements, in which case the rationale is likely to be undermined in implementation.[2]

What we are discussing has been called the "port of entry" problem: How can you enter and become part of a setting in ways that illuminate its features and dynamics? This problem has been discussed best in the anthropological literature. An anthropologist does not decide one day to study an exotic culture and get on an airplane and take off the next. Before going, he or she becomes familiar with whatever has been written about that culture (the beginning of the process of knowing the territory). But before taking off, the anthropologist knows (has been trained to know) that there is no sure-fire guide to understanding the culture; it will appear and be different in important respects from the imagery the literature about it conjured up. (It's not unlike the difference between what an organization chart depicts and how the organization is *experienced*.) On arrival, the initial and most important task for the anthropologist is to select an "informant," someone willing and able sincerely to be informative, to counsel, to prevent the anthropologist from blundering, to suggest whom to avoid and whom to try to get to know. The selection is crucial, which is why some of these studies produce distorted results or have to be regarded as failures. But the anthropologist seeks to understand the culture, not to change it. Gore seeks both to understand *and* to change the culture, and that makes quite a difference, which is why we have emphasized how crucial the selection of coordinators and boundary crossers is. If, to a degree at least, they do not possess the characteristics we described earlier, the process will fail. Understanding the rationale is one thing; having the characteristics to act consistently with it is quite another thing.

We are saying that if you are the vice president, you have to be aware you are starting a network of individuals who you believe have certain things in common. Beyond this, however, is another question: What forums have to exist that not only sustain but enlarge the network? And who will mentor, or mediate, or coordinate the network, formally or informally?

The report (1993a) lays out the strategy in these terms:

> While there are many approaches to promoting organizational culture change, this report focuses on four strategies that explicitly address organizational structure and have successfully changed large bureaucratic organizations in the private and public sectors:
>
> • Streamline headquarters and field structures.
> • Reengineer work processes.
> • Create boundary crossing partnerships.
> • Create self-managing work teams.

These four strategies for transforming organizational structure and culture are interrelated. Implementing one strategy successfully usually involves using the rest [pp. 7–8].

We are told that the devil is in the details, and we quite agree in the sense that the reinventing-government publications do not contain those details that would allow us to conclude that the means-ends problem is being appropriately attacked. What we have been given is a rationale and good intentions—which, like love, are not enough. If we did not expect a spelling out of all the details, we did expect, at the very least, explicit recognition that the coordination and boundary crossing process is akin to a road full of potholes. More correctly, to get to the point of productive resource exchange and boundary crossing and sustain it requires a process that from the start contains the seeds of the alterations you seek to bring out. Change does not start down the road; it starts at the beginning of the road, i.e., with those of status and power who because of their socialization into government are too likely to see "others" as objects of change. The top-down mentality has to be unlearned, which requires creating contexts where it can take place. Refreshing and promising as the reports are, they provide absolutely no indication that the effort will be monitored such that we can learn from hoped-for successes and the unpredictable number of failures.

Reinventing Government in the Eighteenth Century

Although the participants in the constitutional convention of 1787 did not use the vice president's term, their convention is without doubt the best and clearest example of reinventing government in its structural, philosophical, and psychological aspects. The stimulus for that unique event was the recognition of the inadequacies and dangers of the Articles of Confederation. Several things had become apparent. The Articles could not be a basis for forging a nation and protecting it against external enemies. If not superseded, they would centrifugally further separate the states from each other, pit state against state, and make the perception of common interests and actions consistent with those interests difficult if not impossible. The Articles were a weak reed on which to depend for serving and protecting the needs and rights of free people, as well as for ensuring that the voices of people would be heard and heeded. The philosophical-conceptual basis of the Articles of Confederation did not adequately confront the allocation and control of governmental powers, nor why in human history glossing over those issues always led to tyranny, i.e., the needs, rights, and capabilities of people were in the background, not the forefront, of governmental purposes. People existed for those purposes, not vice versa. People were "just" people, servants not participants, passive not active, plodders not creators, dependents not independents. People were "tamed" to conform to governmental purposes; it was inconceivable that people should expect to "tame" government to be servants to the people.

For participants at the 1787 convention, these tasks were not mechanical, a reassembling of parts, a problem in the structure of government. A new structure was, of course, the ultimate goal—but it had to be a structure that would prevent undue sectarian, partisan, and geographical divisiveness, protect individual needs and rights, and be subject to amendment depending on circumstances and the free exercise of the right to vote. The founding fathers were not utopians. They did not believe that individuals were perfect or perfectible; nevertheless, they had a view of the individual's potentials, his ("she" was not yet in the picture!) inalienable rights—a "new" man in a "new" world—that a new structure was preeminently obligated to foster and protect. The 1787 convention did not seek to repair the Articles of Confederation. It started from scratch. The participants were out to prevent what had never been prevented for any extended period in human history: the needs, structure, and style of government taking priority over the needs of the people.

The convention came up with features, two explicit and one implicit, still relevant to today's reinvention of government. The first explicit feature is the concept of the separation of powers, i.e., that the protection of liberty and individual pursuits should be the responsibility of independent arms of government, each with the power to "check and balance" the others. The second and related explicit feature was that these independent arms were in very practical ways dependent on each other; each should be or had to be sensitive to the other two; each in discharging its responsibilities could not ignore the others; each was not a "law unto itself"; and each was in a context of mutuality the purpose of which was to serve the people consistent with law and clearly stated rights and values.

What is implicit in the Constitution—but quite explicit in the proceedings of the convention—is that in the arena of government and politics sectarian-parochial interests are omnipresent, as is the role of "brokering": "You scratch my back, I'll scratch yours," "You do this for me and I'll do that for you." The founding fathers were enamored of the inalienable rights of people, but far less so of the capacity of people to be dispassionate, self-sacrificing, or wise. They did not fear brokering—that went with the territory. They feared a partisanship that subverted the perception of mutuality of interests and goals. There was a difference between principled brokering—best illustrated during the several months of the convention's deliberations—and a partisan brokering of the "zero-sum game" variety: "When I win you lose, there cannot be two winners." If the founding fathers—who, to our knowledge, never used or invoked the concept of principled brokering—saw the actions implied by such a concept as necessary and even inevitable, it still proved impossible to incorporate the concept into the formal document. What they counted on (hoped, really) was that those who were part of government would possess the maturity, statesmanship, and vision to seek to avoid the too-frequent fateful consequences of narrow partisanship in which the general welfare was sacrificed for partisan gain.

Brokering is not the same as coordination, even though it involves issues quite relevant to the coordinating role and its functions. For one thing, the concept of a *broker* is associated with the image of a person who serves as an intermediary between two or more parties seeking to exchange, buy, or sell resources having monetary value and from which exchange the broker receives a fee the size of which depends on the price the parties agree to. *The broker is a partisan; he or she has a vested personal-fiscal interest in the outcome; the broker is not neutral; there is a conflict of interest.* Clearly this is not what the founding fathers would have meant or hoped would be the dominant feature of relationships within and among parts of government and between government and external individuals and groups. But there is another type of broker the founding fathers would have understood and commended: the *honest broker,* a person who seeks an agreement fair to all parties, a person who starts and ends with no power, an informed but selfless individual who seeks to help the parties enlarge or alter their view of their mutual interests. That, of course, describes an ideal—but it is an ideal based on private and public values that were evident during the convention and one that allowed its participants to hope such values would suffuse political relationships in and around the newly created government. If it did not work out that way, if *politics* is used as a pejorative term now as it was then, let us not forget: the founding fathers knew that inventing a new structure of government was one thing, but ensuring that its structure would be powered by an appropriate morality and vision was quite another thing. What they had made explicit depended on the implicit. For government to be responsive and self-correcting required a new structure, but that was a means, not an end.

The founding fathers had no basis for envisioning the steady, dramatic, even fantastic growth in the size of government as well as in the number and size of other private and public institutions. Nevertheless, the explicit and implicit issues with which they coped are identical to those giving rise to today's effort to reinvent government—which is only the latest of many similar efforts, albeit with a more ear-catching label. What these efforts share is a concentration on several interrelated questions: How can existing resources be more creatively and efficiently used? How can they be more responsive to the needs and voices of people whom government was set up to serve? How in an age of bigness can we prevent "parts" from becoming bounded and rigid entities that exist for themselves, unaware or uninterested in or even dismissive of their obligations to the overarching purposes of the "whole"? How do you create and sustain obligation to mutuality and exchange of resources so that the walls between parts are more porous and translucent, thereby diluting the worst features of turfdom? Is there no way by which the centrifugal forces that separate parts from each other can be countered by centripetal forces?

Looking Forward

In a way, the reinventing-government effort is hoisted with its own petard precisely because its rationale and diagnosis are so clearly and refreshingly on target in its call for boundary crossing and productive coordination at the same time that it glosses over (ignores) what this means for implementation. The word *reengineering* occurs frequently in the reports. Well, in regard to boundary crossing and coordination, the word is scary. It sounds too precise for a process better described as *informal*. To achieve the project's goals involves a change in thinking, a change in time perspective, a selection and dependence on certain types of people whose location and characteristics are neither apparent or predictable, the emergence of forums that are a novel blend of the formal and informal, and what we call a creative patience that helps one tolerate the *Sturm und Drang* that is completely predictable in an organization created on the basis of outmoded conceptions of efficiency. The alternative word *messy* is not pejorative in this context; it simply indicates that what we have described has few or none of the features depicted in organization charts. Where the conventional connotations of *messy* are appropriate as descriptors is evident in the many examples the reports give us about organizational craziness and wasted resources. There is a difference between surface messiness and firmly rooted, predictable organizational craziness. The type of organizational messiness to which we refer is a condition one expects to experience before new order can emerge. Any organizational change intended to be systemic can never avoid a period of messiness and disorder—both of which always look to the entrenched bureaucracy like forms of poison or self-inflicted organizational suicide.

In this book, we offer a suggestion that traditional organization theorists assure us is not practical.[3] We believe certain individuals can and should have as their full-time role three informal tasks. The first is constant scanning of the organization to determine where and with whom resource exchange would be fruitful. Because the individuals know the territory and have time to expand that knowledge, that scanning would in principle have no limits. The second task is, again informally, to take steps (not predictable ahead of time) to forge a network of individuals whose self-interests would be furthered by participating in forums devoted to possibilities for resource exchange. When these forums are started and what their characteristics are will vary depending on circumstances and the chemistry of interpersonal relationships. Starting a resource exchange or boundary crossing network cannot be done by the calendar or a manual of instructions. The third task derives from the fact that an organization has commerce with others (individuals or other entities) external to its borders. In the case of the federal government, the Department of Agriculture interacts with, or influences, or is influenced by, other departments. Each department has external, nongovernmental client populations it serves. The task of the coordinators would be to regard such individuals or entities no differently than they would parts of their internal organization.

The coordinating role we recommend is informal, having no explicit powers. This in itself would make it integral to the new paradigm, as the old one has no room for a role that is both informal and essential at the same time. Why the emphasis on *informal*? The answer is simple: there is a world of difference between *wanting to* participate in a resource exchange process and network and *having to* participate. This is especially the case where organizational history and traditions are inimical to new and strange ways of "doing business." What is perturbing in the reinventing-government documents is that while they explicitly call for a change in the organizational culture, there is nothing to suggest a sensitivity to how easy it is for old habits to remain intact, albeit cloaked in the rhetoric of a new style. Indeed, nothing in these documents suggests there might be a justification for a new role that would deal in unconventional ways with the problems of coordination and boundary crossing so well described therein. It is as if conventional leadership, heightened motivation, visions of improvement, and the formation of teams will be sufficiently strong incentives to accomplish the goals inherent in the rationale. We doubt it; our experience and those of others do not permit great expectations. We have seen too many instances where initial enthusiasms get diluted or are extinguished when the implications of change become apparent. Although our sources of information are few, what we have learned about the happenings in the reinventing-government effort provides no basis for optimism. But even if we discount that information, more sadly there is no provision for describing the effort so as to allow anyone to learn anything about what happened and why. We will end up with anecdotes devoid of contexts and the details of process.

There is another reason for describing the coordinating role as we have, and it concerns a factor usually ignored, far more often than not grossly underestimated, but one that gives rise to actions that subvert goals. We refer to *time*. More specifically, we refer to the obvious fact that anyone in a conventional organizational role does not have very much "free time," and many have no such time at all. Everyone is or appears to be very busy. So, if you seek to foster and sustain productive coordination and boundary crossing— and to do it in a way that you hope will spread throughout the organization—it will require a lot of time over and beyond people's other responsibilities. Unless, of course, you approach the task in a narrow, engineering way in which you bring people together, exhort them to collaborate, and assume commonality of purpose and understanding. That almost always has the appearance of appropriate action with the reality of shadow boxing. But if you understand the resource exchange rationale; if, in addition, you understand the *predictable* problems that will be encountered in forging a network consistent with that rationale; if you understand the necessity of having someone who will facilitate and render supportive (not directive) services to the network; that is, if you become clear about these matters, then you need the kind of coordinator we have described. And it is a full-time job! It is not a job someone can do in addition to other responsibilities. It is also not a role for which you can write the usual job description. One of the authors tried to write such a description, but she stopped when it became apparent the description would be several pages long. Do you call that person a coordinator and then have to disabuse people about the lack of authority to coordinate anything or anyone? Do you call the person a facilitator and then have to deal with questions about what facilitation means? Labels are a very mixed blessing; in organizations, their adverse feature is the requirement that they stand for recognizable skills, special knowledge, and concrete responsibilities so that you understand what the person will be visibly doing during the day. The role we have described is hard to label and describe because we have been describing a kind of *person* who has characteristics we have attempted to specify. If there is ambiguity in all this, there is no ambiguity about two things: organizations need this kind of person, and what that person does will fill his or her days.

Organizations cannot tolerate ambiguity or a change process that, relatively speaking, will not pay off in the near term. But the *culture* of organizations cannot be changed quickly. It is theoretically and practically impossible. It is extraordinarily difficult for organizational leaders to confront, let alone understand, why that has to be so, and in large measure that explains why they would have difficulty creating the kind of coordinating role we have

described, i.e., it is an unfamiliar and strange role, and when it will
pay off is neither clear or guaranteed. As one executive said, "You
are describing a loose cannon." If he had understood what we had
said to him, he would have been correct that indeed it was a loose
cannon—but one without firepower.

We do not regard the coordinating role, as we have described
it, as a panacea. We are quite aware that however considerable our
experience, it has been with informal resource exchange networks.
And we are also aware that the coordinating role we describe is not
a recognized role in most formal organizations. What we find
encouraging is that crossing boundaries within and among organizations is an idea that has begun to take hold among theorists and
practitioners. We do not want to exaggerate the momentum and
strength of the recognition. Certainly on the level of conceptual
rationale the idea has gained currency. On the level of implementation, we simply do not have descriptions to judge accomplishments and to increase our understanding of the complexities of
implementation.

Are the conclusions we have drawn based on our experience of
informal networking applicable to the private sector? We believe
they are, and Chapter Six returns to the point to describe several
accounts that appear to answer the question affirmatively. First,
however, let us explore the rationale behind the new paradigm in
detail in Chapters Two through Five.

Notes

1. The rationale is not all that new. Frost, Wakeley, and Ruh
(1974) spell out aspects of it in great detail, and they cite writers and practitioners before them.
2. Nowhere are these points more clearly described than in the
literature on school change. The intractability of schools to
efforts to change them—whether by people internal or external to schools—rivals that of the past efforts to change the
culture of government (Sarason, 1990, 1993b, 1995a, 1996).

3. The most frequent mistake made by those seeking to change an organization is in adopting an unrealistic time perspective. By *unrealistic*, we refer to not facing up to all that we have learned about the complexities of and obstacles to change. To avoid this mistake, the Industrial Areas Foundation (discussed in Chapter Six) has participants spend the first year or so devoting themselves to countless individual meetings and home meetings. There is no flight into community action. The groundwork has to be laid, pivotal individuals located, and issues and priorities clarified and agreed upon. That takes time, but it pays off in results (Rocawich, 1990; Watriss, 1990).

Chapter Two

Redefining Resources

It is axiomatic to the field of economics that resources are limited. However, until relatively recently in American history it was an assertion that the general public was not aware of, or ignored, or dismissed. The American worldview rested on the belief that no social problem was unamenable to solution once there was a national resolve to garner the needed resources to address the problem. The resources existed, they would be forthcoming, but only if there was a national consensus that the problem had to be addressed. The Great Depression mightily called that aspect of our worldview into question, and the consequences of America's ascendancy to super-power status after World War II made it even more difficult for people to continue to believe that this country was a Garden of Eden possessing the resources to deal equitably and effectively with all problems. Today, most people grudgingly find themselves accepting the belief that problems seem infinite while resources are limited. Generally speaking, this change in outlook is reflected in two often-heard statements: "We have to make choices" and "We have to get a bigger bang for our buck." The second statement gives rise to controversy, but not because anyone is opposed to getting a bigger bang for their bucks. What is puzzling is why so many efforts at repairing people's deficiencies and inadequacies—efforts preceded by a good deal of thought and planning—simply fall short of the mark, frequently very far from the mark, sometimes followed by new efforts with equally disheartening results.

Few would disagree that this description captures the way many people feel about the fruits of federal, state, and local programs.

The fact is, issues of quality and effectiveness of outcomes are no less apparent in the private sector. Indeed, it may be that no industry grew faster after World War II than the consulting industry. Attempting to deal with and repair stagnant or failing or troubled companies occupied thousands of people and cost billions of dollars. The consulting industry was and is big business. In any event, during the post–World War II era people's confidence in public and private organizations dramatically lessened, in terms of their purposes, quality, and efficiency.

Long before World War II, the word *bureaucracy* had pejorative connotations. At the core was the feeling that the larger the bureaucracy, the more faceless, puzzling, convoluted, and wasteful it was: wasteful of resources and defeating of the purposes of those whose interests it was to serve. Musicians say about the Beethoven Violin Concerto that it is not for the violin but against it. Whatever the origins in theory and rationalizing justifications of bureaucracy, in practice it is against and not for efficient use of resources. This is why expensive consultants, commissions, and task forces are created to determine where the problems are and to correct them.

When a problem appears to be intractable, it is safe to assume that we are employing, or are unwitting prisoners of, assumptions that are wrong on the whole or in part. In our earlier books (Sarason & Lorentz, 1989; Sarason & others, 1989) we challenged those assumptions on the basis of detailed descriptions stemming from our experience that were informed by a view of coordination and resources quite different from the conventional one. But generalizing from that experience was very problematic; the broad new paradigm had not yet begun to show itself to us, and our experience was with an informal network of individuals each of whom worked in schools or different public or nonprofit agencies in the sprawling arena called "human services." In that arena, coordination within and between agencies and institutions is in practice a foreign concept, except on the level of rhetoric; but our rationale and the particular kind of coordinating role to which it gave rise had proved itself feasible and productive there. Despite that success, it is a substantial jump from the human services arena to today's great formal organizations, which seem to grow ever bigger and harder to coordinate day by day.

Coordination and Resources

One of the chief liberating insights of the new paradigm is that coordination becomes easier if you redefine what it is you are coordinating. The old saying that money is a necessary means of exchange among strangers is useful here, as it reminds us that there have been and are other foundations for resource exchange.

There was a time when the present authors had no hope that what we had learned stood a chance of surfacing among leaders of formal organizations. Several things brought glimmers of hope, however. The first and most influential for us was our discovery of the Scanlon Plan, which had revolutionized union-management relations in some firms in the period immediately after World War II (Frost, Wakeley, & Ruh, 1974). The plan is still in use in a few large and complicated private-sector organizations. There are striking similarities between aspects of the Scanlon Plan and our rationale, although the plan is far more encompassing in that it affects almost everything about an organization. However, although its sponsors are quite aware of the coordination problem, the plan does not speak to it directly or concretely. There is no coordinating *role*, no addressing who is in it, its scope, its functional style. The desired coordination is assumed to be a function of other aspects of the plan, and up to a point that may be the case. The results were impressive, but far less so in the absence of coordinating roles consistent with the plan's emphasis on the importance of a differential view of people's resources regardless of their label and status. The organization chart had hardly changed; there were changes within this or that part of it, but the boundaries among parts were far from permeable. There was no one whose task it was to foster crossing boundaries.

Since reading the Frost, Wakeley, and Ruh book, we have become aware of similar efforts. For example, in the last several decades it became apparent that in studies of human behavior the dominant (but unexamined) emphasis was in the spirit of the medical model, i.e., what was wrong with people, their inadequacies, malfunctioning, maladaptiveness. Few researchers were considering what made people healthy, productive, and satisfied. What were the relationships between these *individual* characteristics and the *social-familial-organizational contexts* these people had experienced or were experiencing? No one was trying to find out. It is the difference between looking at people in terms of what is "wrong" and what is "right" with them. They are very different types of questions, and they have very different practical consequences. What we call the medical model is not without merit, but it is a very narrow way of understanding, conceptualizing, and judging human performance and capacity. In principle, one cannot quarrel with any effort to prevent a pathological condition, be it an individual, organizational, or social one. But focusing—indeed riveting—on the pathological is no substitute for seeking to create and sustain those conditions in which people acquire knowledge, skills, and ways of thinking that nurture and exploit their interests and capacities, in terms of being individually, socially, and organizationally productive. We are reminded here of what a colleague laughingly said to us when we were discussing the difference. "You might want to use the example of my teenage son, who was reciting a litany of what was wrong with the country. When he stopped cataloging the horrors, I asked him if there was *anything* (in his view) right about our country. He was dumbfounded and for once was speechless. He finally had to agree that he was set only to see deficits, which was one of the few times we have been in complete agreement."

It is noteworthy that the efforts that encouraged us are almost exclusively from the private sector. To our knowledge, there is little in the public sector from which one can generate hope, despite an agonizing awareness on the part of almost everyone that in the public sector hoping for a bigger bang for the buck may best be considered an indulgence of fantasy. For example, one could write at length about the scores of volumes that focus on restructuring the federal government, in each of which "better coordination" is center stage. The vice president's Reinventing Government is only the latest example, though it is the one that comes closest to getting a handle on the problems and finding a new way of looking at things. If you wanted to include state and local efforts over the years, the volume you would write would be too heavy to carry. And who would want to read a litany of failures demonstrating that it is by no means difficult, even with the best of intentions, to reinvent a wheel that never worked in the first place?

Resources and Relationships

Sometimes customs and ways of thinking become so embedded in our institutions—seemingly so right, natural, and proper—that we are rendered incapable of considering alternative perceptions and conceptions. This phenomenon is very much in evidence with regard to two sets of ideas, concepts, or assumptions. The first has to do with how we define people as resources, actual or potential. An analogy may be helpful here. People aren't the only resources we tend to define (and, therefore, pigeonhole) in conventional ways. Originally, oil was defined and used very narrowly, in important but very restricted ways, for lighting and lubrication. Then began a process of reexamination and redefinition, of experimentation, that over the years gave rise to a petrochemical industry where the uses of oil are mind-boggling. Similarly, we argue, in and out of organizational living we have an opportunity to redefine and expand the usefulness of our human resources, but we must stop looking at people in the most restricted ways.

The second set of ideas concerns the means by which we seek to develop and employ those resources in ways that both enlarge the individual's perspective and increase the pool of resources available to the institution for accomplishing its mission. Definitions or attributions influence and largely determine actions. We can all point to examples of the negative or adverse consequences of the self-fulfilling prophecy: we define an individual or group as not having certain positive characteristics or capabilities, we act accordingly toward them, and we end up "proving" our definition was valid. That is one way of describing the history of defining blacks, women, handicapped, and old people. What those histories reveal, of course, is that the self-fulfilling prophecy can have positive consequences once the definitions begin to change. Not only do we literally perceive these individuals or groups differently now, but as a society we seek to capitalize on those changed perceptions for their purposes and ours.

That is the point of this book: to discuss, illustrate, and demonstrate how the customary ways societal institutions define the roles of those who work in them are wasteful, inefficient, and ultimately self-defeating for the individual and the organization, requiring periodic "reinventions" that on the surface appear to be productive changes but turn out to be otherwise. This explains why we introduce the 1787 Constitutional Convention early in our book. For one thing, the founding fathers squarely confronted the "part-whole" problem: how states would be related to a central government, and how the parts of government would be related to each other. It may be termed the structural problem. But the resolution of that problem is not comprehensible apart from a more important and fateful set of considerations, which essentially revolved around redefining the capabilities of the population to participate meaningfully in and take responsibility for governance. That fateful redefinition did not take place without controversy. Could the citizenry be given such responsibility? Were they capable of making wise decisions? Would they be able to resist the siren calls of demagogues? Would narrow, or partisan, or sectional self-interest swamp concern for the general welfare? Was not a largely uneducated mass a shaky foundation for efficient and responsible governance, for the preservation of liberty? The founding fathers were quite aware that they were confronting a structural problem, a reinvention that brought to the fore the redefinition problem: what were the people capable of? We are used to hearing about the deserved place of honor to be accorded the Constitution in the history of struggles for individuality. But that document and the structural arrangements it contains should not obscure the no-less-significant redefinition—which more than a few regarded as a gamble—of the capabilities of a people. It is not surprising that the risks involved in redefinition were also seen by the founding fathers in a narrower context. Would those who were in different parts of government be capable of relating to or coordinating with each other in mutually productive ways, or would allegiance to overarching purpose succumb to seamier aspects of "politics"? In other words, the dangers were not only "out there" in the people but also "in here" in the government. Although they recognized the importance of answering the question, it was bypassed. How can parts be meaningfully and productively interconnected? How can one prevent the parts of government from relating to each other in ways that had characterized the relationships among the colonies, and between each colony and the national center, under the Articles of Confederation? How can a mutually enhancing *coordination* of parts be furthered, if not achieved?

Today, in regard to the structure and administration of almost every type of agency, public or private, no word or concept is encountered more frequently than *coordination*. Specifically, what we hear is the question: How can a more productive, creative, *resource enlarging* coordination be achieved and sustained? How can we make the walls between parts less high and more porous? For example, it is not necessary to do a research study in order to assert that in the post–World War II era the number of employment notices for the position of coordinator of this or that mounted steadily, and the rate of increase has been climbing in recent years. If you scrutinize job descriptions, leaving aside conventional and professional labels, coordination is ubiquitous as a job function, frequently the central one. And if, as we have done, you talk with individuals whose primary function is to serve as a coordinator in their work setting, it is hard to avoid the impression that however important their title or function appears to be, achieving desired coordination is a sometime thing. If you talk to those who are the objects of coordination, more often than not you get minilectures on the difference between appearance and reality, between the rhetoric of coordination and the way things really are.

Redefinition Expands the Resource Pool

We said at the beginning of this chapter that resources are always limited. This is both a problem and an opportunity. It is an opportunity in that the recognition of the problem can and should be a spur to examining how our overlearned conceptions and definitions of resources—especially people as resources—exacerbate the problem. For example, imagine that Congress passes legislation mandating that the number of children in a classroom be cut in half, and it even provides money to do so. This, of course, means that many more schools will have to be built. We know how to build schools. But we would need at least twice the number of teachers, and in light of the number of existing teacher preparatory programs it would be impossible to select, educate, and train the number of teachers that would be needed, especially if criteria for quality of personnel (students and faculty) are not to be lowered. The goal is impossible to attain. But to say that it is impossible is *not* to say that we resign ourselves to the way things are. What suffuses the legislation is the conventional imagery of an encapsulated classroom (in an encapsulated school) where a specially trained adult is the sole resource of instruction. As long as you define the classroom in that way, you are licked before you start. Are there resources both within and beyond the school (older students, parents, others in the community) potentially available for contributing to the educational purposes of those served *and* serving? Granted that redefining people as resources is no panacea, the process of redefinition holds out the possibility that resources need not be as limited as they are under the original definition. But that process requires, at the very least, acceptance of the view that in terms of assets, actual and potential, people are more differentiated than is suggested by the labels we pin on them. The point here is that the redefinition process seeks to have and add "value" for all potential participants. It does not start with an organization chart each box of which contains labels narrowly describing the skills of people in that box. It starts with the question: Given what we want to achieve, who may have knowledge, skills, needs, and motivations that can be employed in mutually beneficial ways? Of course, this is the kind of question the teacher in the one-room schoolhouse had to confront, faced as she was by a group of children varying widely in age. She did not define older students as just students; they also had to be teachers.

It is a glimpse of the obvious to say that we live in an age of specialization. Whatever its virtues—and it does have virtues—specialization is a mammoth obstacle to recognizing people as having assets that the labels we give them obscure. The writers of this book are indisputably senior citizens, and we know well that not so long ago women were "just" women, whose place was in the home, or in the secretary's office, or in the classroom (not in the principal's role, let alone the superintendent's). Women in the armed services? Military pilots? Chairman (not chairperson) of the board? Governor? It seemed obvious then that to redefine the capabilities of women, or for women to redefine themselves, was both ridiculous and dangerous. The story today is quite different, for many reasons, but chief among them is that people were *required* to face the redefinition process, i.e., women were not "just" women, they had heretofore unrecognized assets.

Relevant here is what this country faced as a result of the bombing of Pearl Harbor on December 7, 1941, and our entry into World War II. To say that we were unprepared for war is to indulge understatement. Wars in general, and World War II in particular, are instances when societies necessarily *and* willingly engage in the process of redefining people as resources, i.e., when the demands of the war require that many people, in and out of the military, change their accustomed roles, acquire new skills, make dramatic departures from what they had previously done or even imagined. The usual criteria for "who is entitled to do what for whom" are changed. It happened in spades in World War II, which explains in part why millions of veterans took advantage of the GI Bill of Rights: the experience of self-redefinition during the war was capitalized on after the war. As has been discussed elsewhere (Sarason & Lorentz, 1989), the post–World War II years can be appropriately labeled as the era of redefinition of people's roles and assets. It took a war to start the process. Unfortunately, the significance of that process has hardly influenced the ways in which public and private organizations view those who are in them. Why this is so, and how it might in part be remedied, is a central theme in this book. It is one thing to articulate a social and organizational problem. It is quite another to avoid remedial actions that are unreflectively informed by the narrowest of conceptions of available resources, ensuring that limited resources will always stay limited.

The reader does not have to be told that too many people feel their interests and capacities are going unfulfilled, unrecognized, or underutilized. The reasons are many and it is far beyond the purposes of this book to discuss all or most of them. Suffice it to say that much has been learned about the nature and sources of those feelings, although it is also the case that what has been learned has not been taken seriously on the level of policy and action. Far more often than not, it is because there is such agonizing (and understandable) awareness of problems—what is wrong with people and organizations and how to deal with them—that a preventive approach is viewed as a kind of luxury for which time and resources do not exist. When you are dealing daily with problems that are pressing and numerous, you do not look kindly on a preventive way of thinking that does not deal *directly* with those problems, especially if in light of limitations of knowledge, time, and resources you are unable to deal with more than a few of these problems. Put in another way: problems are seemingly limitless, but practical answers are not.

If all of this is understandable, it is at best self-defeating and at worst inexcusable. What we quarrel with is not the necessity, moral and otherwise, to deal with repair but the near-total neglect of a preventive approach, of any effort to promote health, that is not the same as dealing with this or that dysfunction or pathological condition. This is why in this book we examine the issues surrounding coordination: they are issues that allow us to contrast the two radically different ways of thinking and acting. One emphasizes how things should be, the other how things can be. One has failed time and again; the other has a far better track record. One starts with a predetermined conception of what people are capable of and therefore where they belong; the other starts with a far more differentiated conception of people's assets, interests, and needs.

We label the former, which reflects the essence of the old paradigm, the "organization chart mentality"; the other we call the "boundary crossing mentality." Our central theme can be succinctly put this way: how you define resources makes a difference in how seriously you regard prevention as the promotion of individual and organizational health. This book is about coordination in organizations. It is also about how and why that coordination must rest on a conception of the differentiated assets, actual and potential, of those being coordinated. Resources are limited, but they need not be as limited as they are.

Chapter Three

Breaking the Organization Chart Mentality

The typical organization chart has a mechanical flavor. It asserts that parts—human subgroups—are assembled or structured to operate smoothly, to be concerted much as the different instruments of an orchestra are supposed to harmonize. Between and among these organizational parts, bidirectional arrows denote reciprocal influences or responsibilities.

Organization charts are impersonal. They say nothing about people. They assume that those who "people" the parts of the chart will act in intended, smooth, concerted ways. An architectural blueprint is not a building; it is a piece of blue-and-white paper containing drawings intended to conjure up and reflect the intentions of those who commission the building and will live in it. Frequently, of course, when they come to live or work in the building, they find that the imagery they thought was reflected in the blueprint has not been realized. Similarly, organization charts, however complicated and detailed, however much they contain bidirectional arrows to emphasize coordination of parts, in no way guarantee the desired coordination. Indeed, they cannot, if only because they refer to abstract parts and say literally nothing about the realities of human purposes and interactions. A word is not the thing to which it refers, a blueprint is not the building that will be erected, and an organization chart is not what coordination will be in real life.

But organization charts are necessary and important because they attempt to describe relationships and purposes among parts. That is a crucial function when a new organization is being created—a time of good will, enthusiasm, and high hopes, a time when all the predictable problems of coordination are seen as minor issues that will be prevented or overcome by the commitment of the creators to the value and necessity of coordination. However, it seems to be a law of organizational development that not long after the creation of the new setting the need for altering the organization chart becomes apparent—precisely because coordination among and within parts has not been achieved. It may be called restructuring, administrative reorganization, or the pursuit of efficiency, but it is almost always the case that the changes center around coordination—its problems and failures. In these days when mergers and takeovers are daily fare, the issues surrounding coordination are a central focus.

"Let's go back to the drawing board" well conveys the imagery the concept of coordination conjures up: the parts have to be reassembled, the bidirectional arrows have to be altered, the overall structure must be forced to take on a new appearance. It is, of course, true that the chart makers realize (in varying degrees) that the problems of coordination are not independent of the personalities and perspectives of those whose responsibility it is to "act in concert"—to put operational flesh on the skeleton of the chart, to make sure that the bidirectional arrows are reflected appropriately in practice. So it is by no means infrequent that before redesigning the chart, the coordinator (or coordinators) are changed. The problem is diagnosed as one of personalities, not as a conceptual one centering around key questions (How do parts define their assets and responsibilities? How do parts define the assets of adjoining parts? What stands in the way of parts capitalizing on each other's assets as the charts require?). Anyone even faintly familiar with the literature on organizational behavior and development knows how much of it centers around the problematics of coordination, more specifically, the gulf between rhetoric and practice, between how coordinators are supposed to think and act and the ways they do think and act in practice. As more than one coordinator has said, "I know what the organization chart displays. I know the intended rationale. I believe in that rationale. But implementing that rationale is another story."

Why Charts Don't Work

The reasons why charts don't work are many, ranging from the predictable consequences of turfdom to the ideology of professionalism and, of course, to personality factors and style. But what the traditional organization chart implies is that coordination is mandated by some superior agent external to the parts to be coordinated. That is to say, parts are to be coordinated; left to themselves they are not likely to seek coordination. It is precisely those exterior agents whose imagery of coordination is basically mechanical. They are the ones who develop organization charts, who know all the parts, and who convey graphically and in language how and why the parts should be coordinated.

Organization charts never indicate how the predictable problems of coordination may be confronted and handled. The unverbalized assumption seems to be that if you put the parts together and indicate their relationships properly—in a mechanical process that anyone can carry out with sufficient thought—the desired coordination will be realized. So there is no need for intermediary roles or forums to deal with problems. There are, in the jargon, no fail-safe processes, no backup, no self-correcting procedures. Why bother? If the parts are properly made for each other and properly aligned (and the creator is sure that they are), then they *will* function smoothly. So when the parts turn out to be poorly coordinated, the obvious response involves four corrective measures: change the coordinators (if there are any), come up with a new chart, resort to hortatory proclamations about the importance of coordination, or call in outside consultants to identify the problems and recommend solutions. The outside consultant option is especially significant for two reasons. First, the *functions* of the consultant—to observe and diagnose the parts in their relationships—are nowhere in the organization chart. The consultant is a *temporary* intermediary, role, or forum, and when his or her services are completed, as a rule no comparable intermediary function gets added to the organization chart—after all, the assumption goes, the parts have been lubricated and should now function smoothly. Second, though there are times when the consultant's diagnosis essentially challenges explanations in terms of personalities and style and identifies the absence of roles, processes, and forums explicitly intended to dilute or prevent ineffective coordination, it is very rare for an organization to adopt the associated recommendations. In short, the issue is a conceptual one in that the organization is being asked to alter its internal culture—the customs; the emphasis on repair over prevention; the "let's fix it" rather than "let's understand it" reaction; the assumption that "clear lines of authority and responsibility" are an incentive to "clear, direct, candid expression of opinion"; the belief that explicit, formal processes are more important than what is perceived as informal, time-consuming processes; the defining of the assets of people in terms of their narrow labels and assigned roles and not in terms of what they may know or be able to contribute— and these distinctions are not easily accepted within the context of an organization. This resistance is a living example of the limited idea of human resources and the medical model of organizational review. As many organizational consultants can attest, organizations do not warmly embrace—if they embrace at all—conceptions that discernibly depart from their imagery of mechanical assembly of parts; in the abstract they applaud flexibility, but in practice they fear it will be messy. They cannot give up the image of a smoothly running machine.

It is noteworthy that in the post–World War II era many private-sector organizations were literally forced to change how they envisioned charts and how efficient coordination could be achieved. The change went far beyond reassembling parts or looking for solutions in better personnel selection. The role of employees in regard to responsibilities and decision making, the nature of incentives, in-service training and education, forums for expression of opinion (contrasting or otherwise), flexibility in changing and assigning roles, greater willingness to experiment with different ways of confronting problems of coordination, reduced concern with boundaries of parts—these are some of the things private-sector organizations were forced to confront as past ways of thinking took them further down the road to economic disaster. Someone once said that nothing sharpens the mind more than the knowledge that you will be executed tomorrow. The sentiment accounts for the degree of change in many private-sector organizations. We do not overestimate the change, i.e., we do not claim that these organizations, as Lincoln Steffens said of the Soviet Union after visiting it following the 1917 revolution, "I have seen the future and it works." But neither do we want to gloss over the fact that it has been in the private sector that new ways of confronting problems of coordination have been tried. If there is one characteristic in which these innovations are similar, it is in an expanded conception of the assets, actual or potential, of people.

It is quite another story in the public sector. For example, if you were to observe a random sample of private companies in a particular sector, you would be hard put to conclude that they confront and handle coordination problems similarly. Their organization charts would be far from identical and the frequency and severity of coordination problems would also differ greatly. Again, we are not painting a rosy picture but merely calling attention to diversity in organizational cultures. If you were to do a similar study in public organizations—local, or state, or federal, or schools, or nonprofit human services agencies—you would be hard put to avoid concluding that they are amazingly similar in organizational structure, in rationales for that structure, and in the frequency and severity of the coordination problems they encounter. Indeed, if there is anything about which everyone, in or out of these organizations, agrees it is that coordination of parts is not only a ubiquitous problem but an unsolvable one. Why unsolvable? Veteran staff answer with a past history of repeated efforts to get the left hand to know what the right hand is doing. As one person put it, "They not only do not know, they do not want to know, let alone become related to each other. Familiarity breeds contempt."

Why is this so? Veterans in these arenas give two kinds of answers, the first of which explicitly identifies personality factors: people do not have the appropriate desire to act in concert, they want to be left alone to do their thing in their accustomed way, and they are content with their mission and regard the request or demand for coordination as a threat to their organizational identity or as a threat to their self-definition. As this group sees it, coordination is not an opportunity, it is a restriction, a narrowing of scope or alteration of mission. People are the problem. The second most frequent answer is a variant of the first: people tend to be competitive and power-aggrandizing foragers for resources and thus untrustworthy collaborators; they are usually "resource poor" and are upwardly mobile in that they seek to compensate for their deficits in resources by taking from the resources of others, i.e., the poor taking from the rich. In one respect, however, the second answer differs from the first because it implies that the incentives of the system work to produce a zero-sum game regardless of the rhetoric about the virtues of coordination. It is a system that socializes people to become protectors of their turf.

Far from suggesting the imagery of mechanics, these answers conjure up a kind of jungle, the inhabitants of which are constantly scanning for predators. That metaphor may be overdrawn, but it makes the point that in our public institutions coordination is regarded as dangerous and doomed. The history of failed attempts in public institutions to achieve better coordination, use existing resources more efficiently and creatively, and provide more satisfactory services to the public is not, to indulge understatement, an encouraging one.

The Youth Service Bureau: A Case in Point

Youth Service Bureaus were first created in the 1960s and can be found now in hundreds of communities across the country. The idea was to help keep youth from delinquency "by (1) mobilizing community resources to solve youth problems; (2) strengthening existing youth resources and developing new ones; and (3) promoting positive programs to remedy delinquency-breeding conditions" (Norman, 1972, cited in Blumenkrantz, 1992, p. 20). David

Blumenkrantz, who took over one such bureau as the fifth director in less than five years of operation, wrote a thoughtful and revealing book based on his experiences, which can stand as an archetype of the organization chart approach to the world gone wrong. Our discussion is based primarily on that book (Blumenkrantz, 1992), and readers interested in more detail will find it a very interesting resource.

Youth Service Bureaus were established specifically to coordinate and organize existing services, not to provide new ones. Their creators possessed charts depicting their community's existing human services agencies; the new bureau was not only added to that chart but placed in its center with appropriate bidirectional arrows to indicate its coordinating role. Unreflectively, they had changed the chart in accord with the imagery of the mechanical assembly of parts. Someone once said that it is like Moses coming down from Mt. Sinai with new commandments: "Thou shalt coordinate" and "Thou shalt allow thyself to be coordinated." It is an old story in regard to youth services, and it never works; as far back as the early decades of this century the first child guidance clinics and juvenile courts—both of which were explicitly intended to play coordinating roles—were quickly diverted from that purpose (Levine & Levine, 1992).

Blumenkrantz soon came to the unhappy conclusion that the basic assumptions of the Youth Service Bureau were faulty. He writes:

> Norman promoted coordination by delineating three interrelated functions: *service brokerage*, or bridging the service gap by noncoercive referral and follow-up; *resource development*, or filling the service gap by working with the community in developing new resources; and *systems modification*, or having Youth Service Bureaus constructively challenge established institutions that are affecting youth adversely, resorting to political pressure when necessary to ensure that resources and institutions are available and responsive to youths' needs. . . . In fact, there is no evidence that community,

county, state, or federal agencies have now or have ever had any
desire or ability to be coordinated or to work in collaboration. But
this idealistic, global assumption with no basis in reality came to
drive the coordination function of the Youth Service Bureaus. Norman's delineation of a coordination function was, to put the matter
plainly, a disaster. It set the stage for extreme community conflict
[p. 20].

Where Youth Service Bureaus prospered at all, it was by mov-
ing into provision of services that were not already available from
other agencies. When they tried to work through and coordinate
existing agencies, they found the personnel of those agencies react-
ing with bewilderment and hostility, taking the attempt as a reflection on the adequacy of current efforts. At least in Blumenkrantz's
experience, every attempt at interagency communication was
rebuffed. Eventually, he writes, "Coordination and planning gave
way to loose understandings and to arrangements among existing
community institutions and agencies. 'There are enough problems
to go around' was becoming the motto of collaboration. Coordination came to mean 'You do your thing and we'll do our thing, and
let's not get in each other's way.'"

Thousands of directors of public agencies among whose express
purposes is coordination could tell a similar tale. Blumenkrantz
wrote the book toward the end of his ten-year tenure in his position. We note this because the reader of his book may draw the
erroneous conclusion that his difficulty in striving for coordination
stemmed only from the attitudes of autonomous social agencies in
a Connecticut community. That, he has assured us, was not the
case. *Within* bureaus or departments constituting the community's
administrative structure, his efforts at coordination were resisted.

Several features of his account are refreshing. One is his
attempt to understand the present in historical terms. Youth Service Bureaus did not have virgin births, i.e., what Blumenkrantz
experienced was not explainable only in terms of personalities and
their perspectives. The bureaus were created and based on assump-

tions that were, to say the least, unrealistic (hopeful as they were). The societal context of the sixties encouraged people to see troubled youth as poorly served, the repair mentality as self-defeating in its consequences, and the major public services problem as the absence of an agency charged with the responsibility of coordinating relevant services. Much could be accomplished, it was believed, by interrelating public services in ways that increased available resources for purposes of primary and secondary prevention.

When Blumenkrantz took over at his bureau, he was a young man full of hope, good will, and energy, intent on making a contribution to the community and its youth. He believed the job could be done in good part because the chart said it could be done, and he only gradually realized that the task was doomed to founder on the ingrained separateness of the blocks that the pen had so effortlessly joined on the page.

Personal Experience with Youth Services

The authors of this book are senior citizens. We have been witness to and participated in scores of formal efforts to improve coordination and utilization of resources in order to better serve their publics. They included state, local, school, and human services agencies as well as a variety of agency councils whose existence was explicitly geared to coordination of autonomous social agencies. We have been on more committees and advisory councils than we care to count. It is correct to say that in almost all instances, these efforts were either outright failures or had barely discernible effects. Some instances met all of the criteria of a cure exacerbating the disease.

The most egregious example came decades ago, when Connecticut state officials decided to create a Department of Children and Youth Services to bring under one umbrella the many services for children and youth that were scattered all over the state's administrative structure. The new department was "to bring it all together" in one agency so that coordination and improvement of services would be possible. To the commission that recommended the new department, the bottom line was *not* financial but rather improved services. That these existing services were inadequate and uncoordinated no one disputed, i.e., left hands did not know what right hands were doing, but even when they did the result seemed to be an adversarial conflict.

Needless to say, as Blumenkrantz found, the parts that were to be coordinated did not look kindly on becoming boxes in a new and very complicated organization chart. So it was not surprising that when all these parts were put together in what was a large department, all of the predictable obstacles of coordination came to the fore. Since inception, the department has undergone scores of changes in administrative structure, exacerbated by having to incorporate programs mandated by new federal legislation. It is fair to say that parts that heretofore had been uncoordinated largely remain uncoordinated, unless you regard power struggles and competition for status and resources as indicative of coordination. It is a department that was and remains troubled in regard to coordination.

Where to Go Next

The brief discussion of the Department of Children and Youth Services illustrates the key point that coordination problems in defiance of an organization chart occur as often among parts *within* large departments as in relationships between departments. But there is another significance to what we have related.

We have no doubt that the coordination problems in the department could have been handled so as to dilute the negatively charged affective consequences, i.e., handled more sensitively, more smoothly. We in no way consider personal style to be a minor factor. But personal experience and observation force us to conclude that a sensitive, smooth, patient, even charismatic leadership style is not sufficient to develop *and* sustain coordination. What is required in addition is a conception that deals with these questions:

How are participants defining their assets and those of others? What do they regard as their resource deficits and those of others? Can the resources of each compensate for the resource deficits of the other? Is there a basis for resource exchange that not only "plays to" the self-interests of each (i.e., increases the resources of each) but at the same time begins to forge a sense of relatedness, of a community of interests and purposes? If achieving this is not guaranteed by good intentions or personal style, to whom should such a role be given? How can anyone in such a role avoid being caught up in matters of status and power? Can the role be defined so that it is essentially an informal one but, nevertheless, an influential and persuasive one? What should be, what must be, the personal, cognitive-conceptual characteristics of someone in such a "selfless" role, a role that has no conventional, formal power and to which role an increase in power is not sought? Absent such a person or role, absent a forum for discussing the above questions and possibilities, do we resign ourselves to the luck of the draw, i.e., somehow or other the organizational chemistry will avoid at least some of the major, predictable, upsetting obstacles coordination engenders—struggles for turf and resources—with the result that services to people are not as effective as they should be?

No one argues that formal organizations do not require a differentiated structure containing specialized parts and levels of responsibility and authority coordinated to produce a desired product or service, which is what an organization chart is supposed to depict. The significance of an organization chart is less in what it tells us about parts and authority than in the coordination indicated by lines or arrows connecting the display of boxes going both top-down and sideways. A bureaucracy is supposed to be a "rationally" coordinated array of functions, not a collection of fiefdoms concerned only with their perceived functions, where one fiefdom perceives adjoining ones from the standpoint of foreign relations, where the resources of each fiefdom are zealously guarded against invaders or trespassers. We are not saying anything here that readers who have worked in these organizations have not experienced.

Someone summed it up in the phrase "organizational craziness": it makes no sense. Unfortunately, it makes a lot of sense
because it pinpoints where the problem is: a superficial, mechanical, aconceptual understanding of coordination as a process and
goal, as if coordination is only about connecting existing parts of a
whole. What gets obscured is that coordination is not only about
linking resources but, to return to the theme of the previous chapter, *redefining* those resources (people and things) in ways that add
material and personal value to the organization. We are referring
here to more than human relations and communications because
the style, substance, and problems those words suggest are to a significant degree determined by how we define and redefine people
and things as resources.

As long as we view resources in conventionally narrow ways,
employing labels suggesting that people with different labels obviously possess nonoverlapping skills and knowledge, we drastically
limit the assets potentially available and practically usable to us.
Under the conventional way of defining resources, what gets coordinated among boxes is circumscribed in the extreme, with the
added consequence of engendering and exacerbating human relations and communication problems.

The logic undergirding organization charts is deceptively rational in that it conveys the impression—as it explicitly is supposed
to do—that resources will be used in the most productive ways.
That impression, of course, is belied by one of the most predictable features of organizations: they undergo frequent structural-
administrative transformations to achieve better coordination,
using the same implicit logic that is one of the root causes of the
"problem of coordination."

There are other questions, but the ones we raise here serve
the purpose of emphasizing that the ubiquitous problem of coordination is not only one of the personality style and good intentions of the participants but—certainly no less important—also
a conceptual problem centering on the conventional ways we
define (and, therefore, pigeonhole) people as resources. In and out

of organizational living, we define and apply the resources of people in the most restricted ways, and in the case of organizations nothing is more restrictive than the imagery of mechanics conjured up by organization charts containing boxes, lines, and arrows which, however initially necessary and important, nevertheless in practice bypass the conceptual problem: How can the resources signified by a box be defined and used in mutually productive ways with those in adjoining boxes? The imagery of boxes is one of bounded entities each of which contains narrowly defined human and material resources.

In the next chapter, we describe another form of coordination, outside the confines of organization chart boxes. The discussion is based on the particular kind of network in and through which we gained clarity about coordinators and coordination, an ever-changing network of individuals that has endured for two decades, a network comprising people varying widely in age, status, role, and personality. The ever-changing composition of the network is matched only by its unpredictable, percolating, productive effects.

Chapter Four

Coordination

The Origins of a Point of View

This chapter returns to the topic of our earlier books to explore some features, ideas, and problems we have confronted more directly in the intervening years. These concepts now take center stage in our view of the new paradigm of effective organization.

One Coordinator in Action

As in our first two books, the central figure in our story is Mrs. Dewar, a person of means, a member of a family of national visibility, and a woman with no formal professional credentials. She has long been a critic of the tendency to define or regard an individual in terms of conventional labels, which have the explicit effect of ignoring personal-conceptual assets not suggested by those labels and implying that no knowledge, experience, or interests lie beyond the presumed boundaries of competence. Mrs. Dewar is "only" a private citizen. Who is she to tell professionals, agencies, and institutions that perhaps they are overlooking ideas that will increase their resources for serving their clients? Is she not a do-gooder who clearly is ignorant of the complexities and realities of the human services and educational institutions? Mrs. Dewar has always made it her business to highlight hidden resources—by seeking interviews with or telephoning, or writing to, a myriad of officialdom. Over a long life she became very knowledgeable about hospitals, schools, mentoring programs, professional training programs, the legislative-political-public policy arena, social services agencies and councils, and more. She is a self-trained generalist. It is correct to say that she knows the formal and informal workings of her geographical area (and beyond) as few people do. Many people listen to her, few hear her—though in the past two decades the number of people she has helped and influenced has increased dramatically.

More remarkable than Mrs. Dewar's knowledge of agencies, programs, and community issues and problems—and the number of people she has made it her business to know—are several very clear conceptions central to her thinking and actions.

- *The dominant orientation informing what we will call the "human services" is one of repair rather than prevention.* Agencies insist on responding to problems only after they have become just that: problems. What troubles Mrs. Dewar is the almost total lack of discussion about and actions relevant to prevention— by which she means the active promotion of ways of locating and exploiting the interests and capacities of people and matching them complementarily or for mutual benefit with the interests, capacities, and needs of others, thereby increasing the resources available to each. This conception of prevention is not oriented to this or that problem but to the application of people's existing assets for the purpose of building on and exchanging those assets in mutually enhancing ways.

- *Human services professionals tend to perceive the people they are serving in terms of their deficits or pathologies and to ignore their assets.* This perception makes it impossible to build or capitalize on the assets of the community allegedly being served. From Mrs. Dewar's standpoint and experience, almost everyone possesses some personal, cognitive, attitudinal assets that can be starting points in the helping process. Her knowledge of professional training programs makes it clear that the deficit-pathology orientation is a major obstacle to the recognition of the possibilities of the preventive way of thinking.

- *Where entertained at all, the concept of prevention rarely goes beyond the prevention of pathology.* As Mrs. Dewar sees it, problem prevention needs to include the promotion of attitudes, strengths, skills, and knowledge that increase people's options for self-directed action. She regards it as a particular opportunity for the schools—though one rarely taken up—to help students to form "maps" by means of which they can begin to understand, apply, and traverse diverse personal-community "networks" that can further their interest and challenge their capacities. To promote "positive health" means sensitizing students (and people generally) to the ecology of their community—to the people and resources the community contains and the ways in which such knowledge can and should be exploited by each individual in it.

- *People rarely have much idea how their interests interlock with those of others in their community.* Mrs. Dewar's great strength is her work with many and diverse *informal* networks—informal in that they do not have names or boundaries, and none of the people involved saw them as groups having a stated purpose, constitution, or formal means for coordination. If you map any of the networks to which Mrs. Dewar feels she belongs, you find that few of the other members were known or had access to each other until she came on the scene. Her self-appointed task is to determine how the needs and assets of a person—whatever his or her organizational affiliation—can be interrelated and used with those of others in mutually productive ways, i.e., how what one person has or needs can be exchanged for what another person has or needs, and it is her aim to articulate such suggestions or possibilities in the most concrete ways.

Mrs. Dewar is a matchmaker par excellence. As one of these people said, with wonder and praise, "She is without question the most remarkable Hello Dolly when it comes to suggesting and even arranging matches between people who do not know each other but need each other." What deserves emphasis is that Mrs. Dewar is a fount of suggestions, a provider of information, an encourager, an always-available person, a constant scanner and exploiter of her ecology near and far. She never directs, intrudes, or hectors, even though she frequently despairs at how strange the idea is to people that what they have or need can be exchanged for what other people have or need. The networks Mrs. Dewar has built comprise individuals who are formally part of some kind of public or non-profit agency but whose relationship to others in that nameless, unshaped network are informal, although the substance of their relationship frequently influences their thinking and actions in their organizational roles.

The Underlying Concept

None of Mrs. Dewar's actions are comprehensible except when seen as deriving from an amalgam of her conceptions about prevention, how people are defined or define themselves, the nature and use of networks, and the bedrock importance of a coordinating role the aim of which is to bring people together when they cannot accomplish their aims alone but can do so if they join forces. It is a coordinating role without power and one to which accrues no material gain. In that sense, her role does not fit the conventional image of the broker. It is an unpaid, unlabeled role that an undetermined (and undeterminable) number of people, probably not great in number, play in their community. Indeed, it is a high point in Mrs. Dewar's activities when she comes across another Mr. or Mrs. Dewar!

When Vice President Gore's initiative for reinventing government was made public, Mrs. Dewar was galvanized to action. More correctly, she was more than concerned that, as in the past, we would witness another episode of playing around with organization charts, organizational shuffling and rearranging, and the rhetorical encouragement of smoother collaboration, improved service, more efficiency, better coordination. Knowing as she did how zealously parts of organizations protected their turfs, how resistant they were to being coordinated, how they defined a resource as something you controlled and not something you shared with other parts, how rigid the boundaries could be, how competitive parts were with one another—knowing all of this, Mrs. Dewar—being Mrs. Dewar— naturally asked: Will they create a role the sole function of which is to help parts see possibilities for resource exchange which are mutually enhancing, not a role with power but one that alters and enlarges accustomed perception of self-interest? Such a role, she knew, did not exist in formal organizations, but she also knew that in any community there were unpaid individuals productively per- forming such a role in a completely informal way, as she did herself. Were the vice president and his staff aware of what had been writ- ten about and accomplished in that role? Were they aware of what the state of Oregon had developed in and around an approximation of that role? Were they aware of similar efforts in Ohio? Did they understand or even know about formal and informal networks?

Mrs. Dewar tapped into her diverse networks and got in touch with Andy Campbell, one of the vice president's aides. The qual- ity of their telephone conversations is best attested to by his will- ingness to come to her home and meet with her and a handful of members of her resource exchange network. It was quite a meeting, if only because it was obvious to him that the small group had truly long and vast experience with precisely those issues that had led the vice president to initiate the reinvention of government. In addition, he recognized that the group was more than willing to be of whatever help they could render.

For four months, nothing happened. It began to look as though this was one more effort that would bear no fruit. Then Campbell wrote to say that the Office of the Vice President was working with various Oregon officials to build a creative partnership. They were also discussing the possibility of setting up a center to develop people to assume the sort of moderating and brokerage role she'd outlined to him, under the auspices of the National Academy of Sciences.

The letter was a promising beginning, though only a beginning. We do not know if there will be more fruit, but that is not the point of this anecdote.[1] We mention it here as a way of indicating how Mrs. Dewar thinks and acts. She is always looking for ways to form connections depending on people's needs and goals, regardless of how on the surface they are in what seems to be differing roles in very different organizations. She is both scanner and schemer, who sees assets where others see deficits, who sees her role as a suggester and not a director, as a catalytic convener who goes beyond providing information.

The Northern Westchester Resource Network

The Northern Westchester Resource Network comprises individuals varying in age, agency affiliation, educational background, status, and so on; that is, it is heterogeneous. Initially, members came from New York's Westchester County, but the network soon spread so as to include people in several states. It still functions, with Mrs. Dewar as coordinator, but because of her age and health she has been unable to train and supervise a replacement. As a result, the scope of the network is much reduced.

The Northern Westchester Resource Network was born out of a typical web of connections established by Mrs. Dewar. When Dr. Don Davies came to Yale to recover from his tour of duty in Washington as assistant commissioner of education, he was housed with Sarason in Yale's Institution for Social Policy Studies. Mrs. Dewar's acquaintance with Davies led her to read some of Sarason's books, and she promptly asked Davies to arrange a meeting. The two found an immediate confluence of interest in how resources (personal and material) were defined and used, and in positive applications of the concept of prevention as going beyond pathology to promotion of knowledge, skills, and attitudes essential to social, vocational, and intellectual adaptation and maturation.

At about the same time, Dr. Saul Cohen—then at Clark University and later president of Queens College—initiated an action research project on the nature and formation of networks. In short order, Cohen, Sarason, and Mrs. Dewar began a collaboration that initially sought to determine (1) what common ground existed among their different interests and conceptions, (2) whether there was a means of putting them together in mutually productive ways, and (3) where this could be done and who would coordinate the venture. In other words, was there a basis of *resource exchange* that would enable accomplishing more than each could do alone? It was Mrs. Dewar who suggested that we use northern Westchester County, where she had networks that she would endeavor to use for our different purposes. Could we bring those numerous individuals into relationship with each other on precisely the same basis of resource exchange the three of us were forging for ourselves?

We were clear from the beginning about two things relative to network building. First, invitations to an initial meeting would be to individuals who, if they came, would not be representing their formal organizations; they would be there voluntarily (on their own, so to speak) to make of the meeting whatever they wanted. Second, the sole item on the agenda was for the participants to become more knowledgeable about the particular needs and issues confronting them and the others in their working roles. Each of the participants was told who the other participants would be; they were a diverse lot directly or indirectly involved in formal human services, e.g., in county departments, schools, local foundations, community colleges, a residential institution for children, social agencies, and a community council. A few knew each other; some, but not all, knew of each other. The one thing they had in common was that they knew or knew of Mrs. Dewar, a fact that we felt made it likely they would accept the invitation.

The meeting, chaired by Mrs. Dewar, was not a disaster—but it was certainly disconcerting. For one thing, a few people had difficulty expressing their own views and seemed compelled to present the "official" position of their organization, i.e., as if they were representing their organization, a kind of show-and-tell presentation. More than a few were puzzled about the purpose of the meeting. How were they supposed to respond to what others were saying about needs, limited resources, and overwhelmed personnel? How can you share and exchange resources you do not have? How can you think about prevention when you cannot remedy what you are supposed to remedy?

The long and short of it is that we learned again what we already knew. It is extraordinarily difficult for people to think other than in terms of their autonomous, formal organization: its needs, limitation of resources, programs, its perception of competing with others for funding, status, and enhanced recognition. That the organization can engage with others so that its deficits can be partially reduced while its assets serve a similar purpose for another organization without being diverted from its own purposes, allowing each organization to render more and better service, is a possibility alien to thinking, let alone action. If rugged individualism is part of the national rhetoric, it is also part of organization rhetoric. Indeed, it would be surprising if it were otherwise, particularly since funding is such a factor in a competitive existence.

We eventually overcame those obstacles, as described in our previous books. The issues that surfaced in the process are central to the selection and training of coordinators of resource exchange networks, and we address them in more detail in Chapter Five. For our present purposes, it is sufficient to outline the major characteristics of successful network meetings:[2]

- *Groundwork.* Before each meeting, Mrs. Dewar talked individually with each member, asking what the main issue or problem was at the time and gathering suggestions for new items on the agenda. As background, she listed the individuals who would be at the meeting, explained what items were already on the agenda and why, and sketched existing projects that would be reported on. She then sent all the information assembled in these preliminary chats to everyone who planned to attend the meeting.

- *Purpose*. It was made clear (and finally understood) that these were *not* necessarily decision-making meetings, though decisions to undertake projects were made. They were opportunities for people to describe what they were doing and thinking so as to provide a way for others to determine whether a basis for resource exchange should be pursued; if so, dates were made for getting together *after* the meeting.

- *Participation*. Although Mrs. Dewar prepared and chaired the meeting, it was *not* her meeting. Given her style of thinking and acting, she (like everyone else) felt free to point out areas of common interest and need among participants, but in doing so she was (again like the others) "letting her mind go" about "matches" of needs and assets. Rarely, if ever, was the agenda covered in the three-hour session, a half hour of which was for lunch during which members would seek each other out to pursue what one of them perceived as a possibility for interconnecting in some way. Lunch was more than lunch; it was a productive getting together.

- *Reaction*. Summing up the common response, one member said, "These are the most unusual meetings I go to. These are the only times I get to think. I am here because I want to be here, not because I am sent here to represent my organization. Ideas and possibilities get expressed about which I ordinarily would not think at my other meetings. I can talk freely and unofficially and I don't have to be concerned with decisions or matters of policy. They are simply freewheeling, stimulating, and practically helpful affairs. I look forward to them." It is noteworthy that in order to attend these meetings some of the people had to travel up to an hour. Northern Westchester is but a slice of one county, but it is a big county, and although most organizations approved of the network and gave their employees free time to attend meetings, some did not. Some participants had to use their free time and lunch time to attend.

Between these monthly meetings, Mrs. Dewar spent the first week or so talking by phone with all the members to get their reactions to the meeting. She asked if they were pursuing commitments made there, if they saw possibilities for interconnecting with others, and if in light of the substantive reports and discussions at the meeting new people should be invited. She offered to help arrange minimeetings among two or three members when the possibility of mutually enhancing resource exchange had arisen in the main session.

By the end of its first year, the Northern Westchester Resource Network had enlarged to the point where concern was voiced about whether the freewheeling quality of the meetings was endangered. Given the fact that not everyone could come to every meeting, however, the number attending never exceeded thirty-five. But that number masks two facts. First, via the members' own informal and formal networks the Northern Westchester Resource Network became known to scores of people far beyond the county and state, many of whom wanted to learn about how to start and sustain such a network, and a few wanted supervision or help of some kind. Second, here again Mrs. Dewar was pivotal. She would literally spend hours on the phone providing information, putting people into contact with those who could be helpful in their own geographical areas. From time to time, she would meet with a person who sought to become a coordinator, i.e., someone who was eager and willing to travel some distance to talk with her. Over the years, she has played an important role in the lives of these people.

Northern Westchester Resource Network is a misleading label in two respects. First, it was an informal network having no legal or organizational standing; it comprised a motley collection and ever-increasing number of individuals who determined for themselves how, if at all, they could interrelate and exchange resources with others in mutually enhancing ways. Second, as the network grew in numbers and spread geographically, none of the intermittent participants knew (or could know) all those individuals who considered themselves part of it. There was no formal membership list, but each person could learn about any other person via Mrs. Dewar, who was ever alert to the needs of everyone and always scanning her ecology for possible matches. In that respect, she was not only a responder but also an initiator, a veritable fount of suggestions for people to consider, to use or not to use. Mrs. Dewar had no power, but she did have influence. It is not an oversimplification to say that she was perceived as someone who would strive mightily to connect any member with others who had complementary resources, needs, and assets (of one kind or another), i.e., a connection based on what one member said was a "barter economy: you have what I need and I have what you need; is there a basis for a match?"

The Northern Westchester Resource Network began to explore ways to break through the conventional definitions of people and resources. In our work with the network, it became clearer and clearer why those definitions undercut the goals of organizations and of those who work in them, why resources are more limited than they need be, why achieving productive coordination of people and resources has been marked far more by failure than by success, and why it is so difficult to take the obvious seriously. This type of network is not a panacea for the world's ills, nor even a particularly radical idea. As the network member noted, it does have strong overtones of the age-old principle of the barter economy. That principle operates informally in a myriad of ways among strangers and friends, neighbors, and family, but it is well worth paying attention to. In our experience, more often than not it becomes "the tie that binds," i.e., an antidote to narrow self-interest, to a constricted view of the productiveness of the perception of shared purposes, to resistance to recognizing that others, like yourself, have assets that, if exchanged in some way, are mutually enhancing.

The network addressed the universal complaint of public agencies and institutions: adequate resources are lacking to do the assigned task, i.e., to render a high-quality service to some segment of the community. It began to loosen the death grip with which these agencies and institutions clung to the "myth of unlimited resources": somehow, someway it is possible, or should be possible, for society to allocate to each agency the resources it needs to do what society has asked it to do. As a consequence of limited resources, agencies saw themselves in competition for those limited resources—and the substance and style of professional training made it difficult for agency personnel even to consider how autonomous agencies might conceivably exchange resources in mutually productive ways. This perspective generally causes agencies to "know" each other only through the prism of labels, and hence to know little or nothing about agencies whose labels are unrevealing of their programs and assets. The network began to create an ecology of agencies crossing program lines, supplementing the common ecology found in any community, which tends to consist of groupings of similar agencies. These local similar-agency groupings have their virtues as forums for shared interests, but they tend to prevent recognition of the possibility of interconnections outside their narrow field. The Northern Westchester Resource Network provided a mechanism through which apparently very different types of agencies could learn about each other's needs, plans, problems. It takes someone with Mrs. Dewar's way of thinking and scanning to see commonalities where the rest of us see only differences.

The organization of the network keyed into our long-term observation that in their working lives many people come to feel hemmed in, pigeonholed, restricted in their range of experience, desirous of introducing diversity in their work. They feel that they have more to give and to get. This is not to say they are unhappy people, but rather they feel they are capable of being and doing more, of giving and getting more. In many instances, indeed for the bulk of the network participants, these attitudes, feelings, or yearnings were exacerbated by the disparity between the needs of their clients and the resources their agencies had to meet those needs. It was not that they were overworked, though some were; instead, the brute fact was that resources were so limited. Mrs. Dewar's rationale for networks and resource exchange allowed individuals in public agencies to begin to see themselves, others, and their clients from a new perspective, one that enlarged their knowledge and understanding of their community and one that would redefine and build on their assets and those of others. We knew the strength of the obstacles to such a process of redefinition. In our own lives we had personally experienced (more than once) the *Sturm und Drang* of such a process.

When we started the Northern Westchester Resource Network, we were not optimistic about its ability to overcome obstacles to interagency collaboration. Each of us had been part of very different kinds of networks—almost all of which were for purposes of information exchange, not resource exchange—and we were both inexperienced and uncertain about how to proceed in this new field. And our initial steps were frustrating. If we had to identify the single factor that accounts for the network's accomplishments and longevity, it would be that as a consequence of engaging in resource exchange the values of members changed in that they saw the benefits of mutuality as they never had before. They came to have similar values that went beyond any narrow definition of resource exchange, that introduced a new note of sharing into their accustomed ways of seeing themselves and others. As one member said, "I got to know a lot of people through the network, especially the monthly meetings, and what was initially puzzling to me was that the people there seemed to share and reflect a kind of attitude, as if to say that they knew and did things at these meetings that were *special*. The person who had invited me had said that there was something special and that after attending two or three of these meetings I would understand. He was right. There is something special that we share, and it's hard to label or even describe, maybe because it is never a focus, an agenda item. But we certainly see things differently because of these meetings." The comment is from a program director of a community college, who on another occasion said, "Something unusual has to happen for me to skip a meeting. It's not that I gain something from others of direct benefit to my program—that has happened only occasionally—but there is something in the air of those meetings we silently acknowledge and, I would say, treasure. In any one month, I attend scads of meetings, none of which even remotely comes close to the network meetings. To everyone at those meetings, the world simply looks different and less discouraging."

Rosabeth Kanter (1994, 1995) observed a phenomenon very similar to what this person was trying to articulate. In newly formed business alliances she had observed around the world, she described situations where the participants came to share values not ostensibly the purpose of the alliance, i.e., they came to see themselves, others, and their working world differently. (Chapter Six returns to Kanter's work in more detail.) A Supreme Court justice once said that he could not define pornography, but he sure knew when he saw it. Similarly, it is hard to define the values the network members came to share, but those values had an almost palpable presence for the network members—including the authors of this book, for whom those meetings were the highlights of the month's activities, highlights they had not predicted or heretofore experienced in the myriad of groups of which they had been part. We are not trying to convey the impression that these meetings had a Camelot quality, as if everything was sweetness and light, there were no procedural potholes, and no problems of personality style; or that the process of giving and taking, of arranging matches, had a well-oiled, mechanical quality. Rather, always in the background was the shared sense that there was something special about what these meetings signified, a shared sense that was the interpersonal glue keeping us together.

Network Growth and Development

What we have thus far said is prologue to issues we did not anticipate, a direct consequence of the growth of our network, both in terms of numbers and geographical spread. A year after the network began, it became obvious that the time demands of the coordinator's role were more than Mrs. Dewar could or should be expected to handle, even though she had no formal employment and was not seeking it. In addition, it was no less obvious that if anything happened to her, the continuation of the network was endangered. Could we find someone who could share that coordinating role with her? What are the characteristics such a person should possess? How do you find and develop such a person? From a practical standpoint there was another issue that was far more serious, thorny, and clearly fateful, not for us, as we shall soon indicate, but for anyone anywhere who desired to be a coordinator like Mrs. Dewar. Simply put, Mrs. Dewar was a woman of independent means who, along with her willingness to give generously of her time, also provided money for the lunches in the middle of each meeting—interludes that were both enjoyable as well as interpersonally and intellectually productive, and catalytic in regard to possibilities of resource exchanges and projects including groups of members. There were expenses for telephone and mailings of agendas and a good deal of information of general interest as well as information relevant to individual members and those subgroups seeking to determine how they could interconnect their programs, i.e., give to and get from each other. In any one year, Mrs. Dewar's contributions probably did not exceed $5,000, a negligible amount given her resources. But she was giving her time for nothing! Where do you find someone like her, able and willing to share the burden, someone with her knowledge of the local and larger communities and contacts within them? We believed then, as we do now, that there were individuals in the community who in very restricted, informal ways—in their neighborhoods and friendship or family networks—thought and acted like Mrs. Dewar. But those networks did not consist, as ours did, of individuals working in different roles in diverse public agencies and institutions. Besides, even if we could locate such individuals, the task of preparing any one of them for the role would for an indeterminate period require all of Mrs. Dewar's time and more, even assuming that the process of selection, training, and supervision went smoothly, which, of course, we knew to be an unrealistic assumption.

Mrs. Dewar was prepared financially to underwrite a second coordinator. What about members of the network? Were there not some of them who could play such a role? In theory the answer was in the affirmative, and clearly so. In reality, the answer was no. Each member of the network was a highly trained, full-time professional employee of a public agency or institution of some kind, i.e., in a conventional, respected career. None of them could be expected to make a dramatic "career change" into a future of obvious uncertainties, financial and professional. However much they derived satisfactions and benefits from being in the network, they understandably recoiled at the idea of dramatically changing their work roles.

As we emphasized earlier, each member attended as an individual, not as an agency representative, although whatever benefits the member derived from being in the network were also benefits to their agencies. Although these benefits became known to the agencies, who also became quite supportive of the participation of their respective staff members, we were assured that it was completely unrealistic to expect that any agency would give "release time" to a staff member to play a major coordinating role or that the agencies in combination would be willing (or from their standpoint financially able) to create and underwrite such a role. So, despite the fact that the network had demonstrated to the satisfaction of these agencies that its rationale and accomplishments were productive, it could not occur to them or their self-interest to create, develop, or support the Mrs. Dewar kind of coordinating role. This was no surprise to us because the absence of such a role among autonomous, tradition-bound agencies was the reason this network was started in the first place.

If we were not surprised, however, we were certainly disappointed. It was not easy to confront the fact that our rationale was literally alien to the tradition and ideology of formal organizations, i.e., they cannot conceive of a role *within* their organization or *among* organizations that could or should be basically independent, without formal power, and yet with the potential for increasing organization assets. As a management theorist and consultant said to one of us, "You are describing a role that has an oxymoronic quality . . . a role the organization cannot and should not control. Where do you put that role in an organization chart, and how on earth do you write a job description? It's like being a university professor who has one of those distinguished chairs which frees them from all teaching responsibilities so that they can do what they can presumably best do for the glory of the university. It is one of those roaming, free-floating roles that, aside from a few universities, simply does not exist in any formal organization I know." That person was right about "could and should not control" in the usual sense. No one controlled Mrs. Dewar and she controlled nobody, a fact that every new member to the network found strange and inexplicable. Why was she doing what she was doing? What was the payoff for her? What kept it and her going? What was her background? Where did her ideas come from? How did she come to know so much and so many people?

The theorist and consultant was right in saying that formal organizations do not know how to incorporate a Mrs. Dewar into their organizational charts, assuming that the idea could even occur to them. But he knew one other thing extraordinarily well: his livelihood was derived from organizations in the public and private sectors that used his services to help cope with problems many of which (though not all) contained all of the issues of "poor coordination" among parts, programs, resources, and clients. He also knew he was a "repairer" of problems for which the rate of success was predictably modest. When so-called organizational experts dismiss the Mrs. Dewar role as unfeasible, much of their instinctive opposition may stem from the unconscious (or maybe conscious) realization that their own ecological niche would offer less nourishment if organizations were capable of coordinating themselves.

Personal Responses to the Network

For the purposes of this chapter, we asked several of the members of our network briefly to describe the ways in which their participation influenced them. In making our request, we asked them to be as concrete as possible. We present lightly edited versions of two of the responses here.

The Northern Westchester Resource Network: A Legacy
by Joan Barickman

I took my first job teaching in a public school twenty years ago. Right away, I knew one of my first classes was going to be problematic. My eleventh-grade general English met right after lunch. Most of them were exhausted by the time they got to my classroom because they'd spent a long morning out of the district at the technical school. Besides, a number of them had not had successful experiences with English before. It was a big class, twenty-seven students. Alone, I really couldn't meet their needs and I struggled along, feeling inadequate.

Midyear, my new principal suggested I might like to get involved with the Northern Westchester Resource Network. He really didn't have anything particular in mind, certainly not the progress of that particular class; he just believed in "networking."

The network coordinator (Richard Sussman), however, did have something particular in mind: five students from an urban problems class in our high school had been doing a teaching project in one of our elementary schools; the network coordinator wanted me and my general English class to evaluate the project. His goal, of course, was to enable the district to assess the effectiveness of the urban problems teaching project without hiring an outside evaluator.

I agreed and I started that unit in my class by describing to my students the project and what an urban problems evaluation would entail. Then I asked them to list what they thought they needed to learn before they could complete the job. Together we developed these questions:

- What are the goals of the urban problems project?
- How do professionals write questionnaires?

- Are there different developmental, language, and interest levels to consider when we talk to the different groups: children, peers, teachers, principals?

- How do we deal with a subject who is timid, aggressive, or otherwise reticent?

- How should we organize ninety children to interview?

- What are the characteristics of a "publishable" report?

- How do we present data so that it is clear, accurate, and objective (not praise or blame)?

These questions became the curriculum guide for the rest of the unit. Some of our activities were not conventional English. We used "micro teaching" to improve our questionnaires and interview techniques. We listened to tapes of children, teenagers, and adults telling the same story and compared their language and thinking patterns. One group of students read *Between Parent and Child* and wrote a "Guide to Talking with Children." We also reviewed the *Writers Guide* and developed a checklist for publishable writing; so we had conventional lessons on the "sticky" aspects of writing, such as semicolons and dashes. The outcome was a thorough, polished assessment of the urban studies project.

About 80 percent of the students thought the project improved their writing and speaking; Terry, one of the students, said, "I think that it did help me learn English. I learned that different ages talk in different ways. A little kid doesn't talk the way an adult does." I agreed with Terry. I saw evidence in their work that the students understood different language levels. They also demonstrated knowledge of difficult writing concepts such as audience, ambiguity, and implication. They used a variety of written forms such as the research paper, news article, descriptive essay, and opinion paper correctly.

Until the day the principal mentioned it, I'd never heard of a network. After he left, I found myself involved with a coalition of dynamic people from diverse backgrounds, who met regularly to share projects and find ways to trade resources to meet their individual goals. Since then, I haven't had the luxury of an already-formed network, but I do have a network legacy.

The most obvious piece of that legacy is that I now can see my entire environment as an informal resource network. For example, this year Hispanic Outreach received a grant to give free English lessons at the public libraries, but they were having trouble getting recent Latino immigrants involved in the program. Why couldn't high school "global studies" students study the local Latino community and do an advertising campaign for the literacy program? . . . or what about the recent situation when the school needed a VCR? Well, the Drug Abuse Prevention Council wanted to put on a series of programs for parents and couldn't afford several guest speakers. Couldn't the council give the VCR to the school in exchange for a series of educational tapes, written and performed by a drama class? Both of those trades have worked for me in the last year.

Seeing resources differently, however, is only a small part of the effect which the network project has had on my teaching. Even more important is the way it has helped me restructure my curriculum. The students in that eleventh-grade class wrote two reports: one was the evaluation of the urban studies project; the other was an evaluation of our participation. In the second, most of the students commented favorably on the changes in the classroom hierarchy: "Mrs. Barickman worked pretty much as an equal and she relied on our judgment about the questionnaires, interviews and writing." Jeff, another student, said "I think she [Mrs. Barickman] was trying to learn just as much as we were from this project." The change in my role from boss to collaborator empowered students. Most students also felt they were collaborating with one another rather than competing: "Everyone did something and it turned out good. Everyone did it well." "That is the only one time the whole class did something together and it worked out."

All the resources in the world and all the feelings of success and accomplishment in school are irrelevant, however, if schools do not meet their ultimate goal: to enable young people to become responsible, independent adults capable of fulfillment and growth. How better to teach them to be adults and assess their abilities than to involve them with adults in the community? As one of the students, Chris, said, "I think this project is a good thing to do because it involves other people besides the class. This is very different because we are finally getting out and doing something that is entirely new to us." The project itself was real; students were actually doing what adults do. Today, we would call this project and method "authentic assessment."

Through the urban studies evaluation project and other network projects, I learned to ask four essential questions before I organize every course or unit:

1. What should my students be able to do when they finish this course or unit?

2. What project or activity should they do at the end of the unit to demonstrate their abilities?

3. What resources exist in the larger world that will help me teach them?

4. What classroom activities should we do to enable students to acquire the skills, attitudes, and knowledge necessary to accomplish the goals?

Book Talk Dinners developed from my answers to these four questions in literature. . . . Each spring, there is a series of five dinners; each focuses on one book. This year, we are reading *Annie John*, *Of Mice and Men*, *In the Night Kitchen*, *Fahrenheit 451*, and *The Crucible*. We invite a few community members (who love to come and wait eagerly for invitations). Our cooking class prepares an elegant dinner (suited to the book) and the students and adults share an evening of dinner and literary discussion.

The students' performances are assessed holistically by volunteer community members, based on a set of specific standards. The discussions are videotaped and the videotapes become part of the students' final English portfolios. These portfolios are recognized by the New York State Education Department as viable alternatives to the Regents' exams. In fact, our portfolios are disseminated across the state as models of authentic assessment—demonstrations of how students can be assessed on their capacity to do what educated adults must do. . . .

Book Talks are a small example of the legacy the Northern Westchester Resource Network gave me and my students. However, that legacy reaches further. I now teach at our district alternative school, the Academic Community for Educational Success. The Academic Community was founded on the basic principles of the network: sharing resources and goals; empowering students and teachers; involving students, teachers, and community members in common endeavors; and authentic activities and assessments. Over the years, students and teachers worked with literally hundreds of other people in the community. The school itself is run collaboratively by students and teachers, based on a student-written *Constitution*, contract, and code of laws. Together the entire community makes decisions about organization, curriculum, and admissions. The school has become a model of sharing resources, collaborative learning, cooperative student-teacher government, and authentic assessments.

Terry, Chris, and Jeff are now in their mid-thirties. They all still live in my town. Actually, I'm living in Chris's house; we bought it from his family many years ago. Terry works at the market where I buy vegetables; Jeff is an officer in the police department just across the road from our alternative school. I'm acutely conscious that they are now adults in our culture, as are the many other students I have taught. Have they become responsible, independent adults capable of fulfillment and growth? I really don't know Terry, Chris, and Jeff that well any more; but I hope that their experience with the network twenty years ago helped them to keep the attitudes that Chris expressed when he said back then, "I will really try my best to make this project come through for me and everybody else in this class. I'm really looking forward to it."

Network and Collaboration in the Public Sector: Personal Account and Practical Applications
by Toni Colarini (executive director of the Westchester County Youth Bureau, 1988–1995)

I became involved in network activities prior to my appointment as executive director of the Youth Bureau. I participated as Youth Bureau liaison to a project that analyzed census data and that became known as the *Perspectives on Westchester* series. We (the Youth Bureau) worked together with City University of New York (CUNY) Graduate Center and a social service planning agency, the Westchester Community Service Council (WCSC), and the Northern Westchester Resource Network, which was under WCSC aegis. I participated in a number of planning meetings with CUNY Graduate Center administrators and professors to involve students. We defined research needs. The network had purposely brought together active policy making administrators from Westchester together with researchers (both professors and graduate students) in three universities—CUNY, Queens College, and Bank Street College—so as to influence each other. Researchers took their cues from what communities clearly needed to know so that policymakers would be guided by the research which they had helped to instigate.

The Community Service Council, until taken over by the United Way, provided the analyses of the census for all populations. The Youth Bureau extracted for its purposes issues that concerned youth and their families. It wasn't simply a university saying "we want our students to do research and we have chosen Westchester as a place to do it and now we are going to impose our system on Westchester." It was a process of defining a problem and defining a need through a joint process. The impact of the research reports was tremendous. They became the foundation for planning programs, for grant applications, and for defining the needs of children by both public and nonprofit agencies for the 1980s because until we had another census report in 1990, the *Perspectives on Westchester* series provided the only major planning framework for children's services.

During the 1990s collaborative projects continued based on the earlier network activities and resulted in the *Westchester Children's Data Book* in 1993. The name *Westchester Children's Data Book* was modeled on others that had been funded by the Annie E. Casey Foundation on a nationwide basis. So the project became identified as the *Westchester Children's Data Book* with the following partners: the Westchester Community Foundation, Pace University, the Youth Bureau, and the Westchester Children's Association. These data analyses became the foundation for grants and planning during the 1990s. Pace University was the educational arm; they had established the Children's Institute. They contributed students, professors, and interns, and this was a replication of the earlier network model for action research.

To make collaboration work, a network coordinator ascertains from members what needs are their priorities. He or she groups members according to needs and may have minimeetings before a general meeting. When the general membership is gathered, resources are found to add to each project group and advance the purposes of the individual members, their agencies, and the community good. Over time, membership produces different sets of needs, which lead to different services or projects, different reports or different policies. . . .

As a further result of Westchester Resource Network activities, the Youth Bureau funded a consortium program for youth employment, which has become a model for other collaborative contracts. Through the network, we were introduced to Brett Halverson and his work at the Bank Street School Jobs for the Future Program. The Youth Bureau determined that we would implement this program with his consultative and training support. At the initial bidders conference, a group of agencies came together with the expectation of competing against each other. By the end of the meeting a group came together as collaborators and the Consortium for Youth was born. While the employment readiness curriculum continues to evolve over time, the collaborative includes a group of employment and social service agency staff where expertise is in preemployment readiness activities and who then provide targeted services in a highly coordinated way so that youth who were previously unemployable can be successful. This consortium continues to grow, change, expand, and establish training sites across the county. The success of the program has spread so the training cycle may be in one community one time, a group home or residential facility the next time, or a community center after that. Movement is based on who needs training and who is falling through the cracks—youth needing employment readiness training and placement but usually not eligible or ready for other governing programs.

At one point the Youth Bureau had no way of funding a collaboration, but, as with most problems, we found the solution and have created structures to fund collaboratives. We fund one agency to be the leader and then that agency sets up subcontracts with all the collaborating participants. This requires collaborators to sit down and establish contracts for what they are going to do, including expectations and outcomes; it is a performance agreement. So we actually have more collaborative projects going on now. In fact, collaboration is the process of choice for the "Invest-In-Kids" Fund program, which funds youth development programs with county tax levy dollars. All of the projects of the Invest-In-Kids Fund have some form of collaboration as the process to reach defined outcomes. Collaboration and collaborative programs can be promoted by the funding source in requests-for-proposals. In other words, public policy can and should include a mechanism for collaborative planning and activity with a defined coordinator's role as a necessary element to qualify for funding. When an agency prepares a proposal it must describe the mission, the key members of a group who will collaborate to achieve the mission, and the coordinator who will keep it all together. The people who are psychologically ready to coordinate the collaboration, or who have been trained, will have better programs. It really is a skill to be an effective collaborator, coordinator, or facilitator, and that makes or breaks the program.

A particularly successful collaboration, cited by the National Association of Counties' *1995 Best Practices Guide for Children's*

Programs, responded to the needs of Westchester's Persons in Need of Supervision program (PINS). The director of the Youth Bureau coordinated the program and built a collaboration among criminal justice agencies, school officials, and community groups. This program (PINS Adjustment Services) is a collaborative system of services whereby youth who would ordinarily go straight to Family Court for being truant or unsupervised now go through assessment and preventive service delivery processes. The program components are constantly monitored and discussed within a network planning committee structure. The net result has been that the program has documented savings and cost benefits. After considering yearly program expenses, at least $1 million per year is saved in the cost of residential placement of these youngsters, and this is the direct result of the program. This collaboration works for prevention and positive youth development.

This strategy for the PINS program was fostered by a state level mandate for collaboration. New York State provided little seed money but they told counties whom to include in the planning process. The coordinator facilitated the meetings at which the group decided the core needs and how to address them. This has resulted in major systems change. New York State has noted that this program is one of the best in the State of New York. It could not have been accomplished without strong leadership that promoted collaboration. . . .

My experience suggests that resource exchange collaboration provides the means to respond to a variety of needs: research needs, education needs, service delivery needs, and funding needs. Piecing together a collaboration is simplified if you are willing to acknowledge that you or the service you represent cannot provide everything, but if you bring a group together you can add service value to your own and to the other services.

Attitude is an issue that you still deal with at the beginning of every new collaboration. The first issue is a "what's in it for me" and this is usually in terms of dollars and cents. Maybe there isn't a lot of money but perhaps there is an added client pool. If we consider that the bottom line is service delivery to a client pool, then maybe there is something in it for me in terms of service delivery to a population that needs it. We have potential of adding value to existing services because everyone benefits from the resources of the combination of participants.

In establishing a collaborative, it makes sense to ask an opponent or two to participate in the early stages—the ones that you think are the most resistant to the program's becoming operational. The concept of cognitive dissonance comes into play. Cognitive dissonance suggests that the more you invest in something, the more worthwhile, the more valuable you think it is. So your opposition, through participation in the collaborative process, become program advocates over time.

Networking expands your terrain well outside of one county. Threads of interests and projects leap boundaries and raise the phone bill. I have described the impact of network activities that continue and increase day by day. The examples I have presented are suggestions for use and application by people in the public sector. *Coordination* and *collaboration* are too often buzzwords empty of meaning and even intent. Real coordination requires changes in attitudes and ways of using and combining resources.

Conclusion

Mrs. Dewar and the Northern Westchester Resource Network show that interagency coordination is possible. Their techniques are hardly a breakthrough in methodology; mutually beneficial exchanges of value for value date back to the earliest hunter-gatherer societies and are practiced to this day by lawyers and plumbers and others in all walks of life. Nonetheless, organizational structures pose serious obstacles to comprehending the rationale and implementing and sustaining actions consistent with it. These problems pervade the public sector, and the strength of obstacles in the private sector is similar if not identical—and so, as illustrated in Chapter Six, is the strength of collaboration when it can be applied. In recent decades rationales very similar to ours have taken hold in the private sector in foreign countries as well as in ours; red ink and the fear of extinction can be potent stimuli to new ways of thinking.

Where, how, and to what extent our conception of a coordinator can be applicable *within and among* formal organizations, public or private, are not issues we shall attempt to resolve in any definite way. There have been a surfeit of conceptions about coordination proclaimed as "solutions." What we do feel secure in saying is that our rationale addresses in a distinctive way several questions ordinarily not seen in relation to each other: Within organizations having parts, how do you locate and employ the strengths of individuals to increase the assets available to those parts in mutually enhancing ways? Between formal organizations, how do you locate strengths that add to their assets and promote their purposes in mutually beneficial ways? Are there ways by which the predictable problems of forging interconnectedness can, in part at least, be diluted or overcome? What are or should be the characteristics of individuals whose role it is to see possibilities for interconnectedness and to create and sustain forums where those possibilities can surface and be discussed? These are thorny questions and may be seen by some as castles in the air because the questions assume that those responsible for the policies of their organizations will support a role and rationale heretofore foreign to them. To such critics or skeptics, our reply has several parts. First, we have demonstrated to our satisfaction and to that of many others that our rationale is feasible and productive on an informal basis. Second, once an individual grasps the rationale and acts consistently on it, castles in the air take on an earthy, practical, personal reality. Third, no one in our network, and no one in the networks spawned by ours, doubts the practical significance of our rationale for the coordinating role within their own, and between relevant, organizations. Fourth, as we indicated earlier and shall discuss later, there is more than a little evidence from the private sector that rationales similar to ours have taken hold here and there on the basis of sheer self-interest.

This last point deserves emphasis: our rationale plays to self-interests inexpensively.

In the next chapter we address the characteristics of individuals whose role it is to see possibilities for interconnectedness and to create and sustain forums where those possibilities can surface and be discussed. These intellectual, cognitive, and personality characteristics are crucial to the coordinating role. To the extent we can gain clarity about the characteristics and their combination, we gain clarity about how the role can contribute to the assets and purposes of organizations. It also clarifies what is involved in locating, selecting, and developing such individuals. As we shall see, we are dealing as much with self-selection as selection by others.

Notes

1. As noted in Chapter One, we fear that the Reinventing Government program is unlikely to develop an effective coordinating role. From working documents made available to us, they appear to have a conception of a coordinator that bears little relationship to ours.
2. For the reader who wishes a detailed description of these meetings, our earlier books and especially Thompson's dissertation (1985) will be very helpful.

Chapter Five

The Coordinator's Rationale

Cognitive and Stylistic Characteristics

The match between a person and the coordinating role requires far more than a high level of motivation to undertake the role. This is, of course, the common condition of human endeavor: not all physicians should be treating patients, not all teachers should be teaching, not all managers should be managing, and not all leaders should be leading, despite their strong motivation to be in such roles. The point, as obvious as it is too frequently ignored, was made clear by Freedman (1993) in regard to adult mentors of young people. In the area of personnel selection, there is a maxim that if you know how to select, you have licked at least 50 percent of the training problem. Motivation is important, a necessary but far from sufficient criterion for assuming a particular role.

We learned the lesson the hard way in selecting and training network coordinators, almost all of whom were self-selected, i.e., they had heard about our network or read our books. Part of our difficulty was the strength of *our* motivation to select or train or advise individuals who "bought" our rationale, who were eager to do what Mrs. Dewar did. The difficulty was that we were learning as we went along and did not know how to weight other crucial characteristics. We are reminded here of the decade of the turbulent sixties, when every major societal institution was an object of militant criticism and many individuals sought to become "change agents." Their motivation was both strong and exemplary, but they lacked many other characteristics the role required, with the result that their accomplishments were slight, sometimes counterproductive, and their disillusionment personally painful. All of this is by way of saying that the coordinating role we are describing is not for everyone who finds it interesting, challenging, novel, and productive.

Background

In the previous chapter, and in far greater detail in our earlier books, we have attempted to present a rationale for a particular kind of coordinating role. The rationale was derived and developed through creating and sustaining an informal resource exchange network. By informal, we mean that although the network had a name, it had no legal or corporate status, appointed director, boundaries, or written or agreed-upon rules and regulations about participation and procedure. It had movers and shakers (e.g., Mrs. Dewar and several others), but whether anyone else "moved or shook" was unpredictable: what members thought at the beginning of a meeting was not a good predictor of their thinking at the end of a meeting that ran three or more hours.

We created the network as much to test our rationale for resource exchange as to gain personal experience about the coordinating role. As time went on and we and others became convinced about the potential of the role for public and private organizations, it became obvious that it was our obligation to understand better the characteristics of a person who would be in such a role. We are more or less stuck with the label *coordinator* to describe the incumbent of the role—even though that word engenders an image of someone who is empowered, who has authority to mandate or require direct interconnectedness among parts of an organization. That such a role is necessary goes without saying. We are in no way partisan to the view of authority or power as inherently counterproductive. But we have to state the obvious: in formal organizations such conventional, necessary roles achieve their stated purposes very rarely, and they rarely tap into the potentials for building on existing assets or strengths in the different parts being coordinated. The kind of coordinator we have described is no substitute for the conventional one. Their goals may (and ideally should) be similar, in rhetoric at least, but their means, status, and perspectives are not similar at all, certainly not in practice. So in the following discussion we ask the reader to keep in mind we will be describing the ideal characteristics of a person in a unique coordinating role, one that does not exist in formal organizations but should exist there, a role whose time has come if only because in an inchoate or unfocused way increasing numbers of people are beginning to accept and adapt to the brute fact that resources are, as they have always been, limited, and one way of adapting is to redefine people as resources—as assets—not as "one person, one function" units.

We also have to ask the reader to keep in mind that we will be describing a *combination* of characteristics any one of which is possessed by many people but the combination of which is possessed by far fewer. Of course, this makes locating and selecting such a person no easy matter. And it also raises questions about how to develop people for such a role. It is for these reasons (among others) that we have said that we do not advocate what we do in the spirit of a panacea. If in our hearts we are convinced that our rationale has weathered the challenge of practical application, we are aware that by going from the informal arena of working relationships into formal public and private organizations we will confirm the maxim "problem creation through problem solution." Much of what we advocate today was not in our heads when we started our network; we learned as we went along.

For example, when we started we unreflectively assumed that the coordinating role we conceptualized required a resource exchange network, i.e., a mechanism by means of which a coordinator could bring people into relationship with each other. That is to say, the coordinator would be both convener and facilitator. Then we heard about, visited, and studied the late Daphne Krause, head of the Minneapolis Age and Opportunity Center, an agency that achieved semilegendary status in the area of service to older people. Intellectually and in many other ways, she and Mrs. Dewar were twins. However, unlike Mrs. Dewar, Daphne Krause was head

of a large and formal nonprofit agency, and her sole task was to
make services available to several thousand senior citizens as inexpensively and conveniently as possible. But like Mrs. Dewar, she
knew her local scene (and the relevant Washington one) like the
palm of her hand, and no one had to give her lessons about the values and principles of resource exchange. "What does X have that
my senior citizens need, and what do I have or what can I do that
will benefit X?" Such thinking was second nature to her, as it was
to Mrs. Dewar. Where individual or agency X was aware of what
was lacking, Daphne Krause paid attention to assets. The long and
short of it was that Daphne Krause had resource exchange relationships with a local hospital, many state agencies, even more
social agencies, and scores of restaurants. The restaurant relationship encapsulates her way of thinking. If the restaurant agreed during certain hours of the morning and afternoon to discernibly
reduce its prices for the agency's clients, she could promise (but not
guarantee) that their restaurant would not be nearly empty during
those hours. It worked. Also, when she found out (she was always
finding out!) that one of the leading hospitals had a lower occupancy rate than it required, she made a "deal": If the hospital would
accept her clients who were at or near the poverty level and would
charge no more than what the local department of welfare paid—
no questions asked, no differential treatment—she guaranteed that
the occupancy rate would rise; if not, the deal was off. It worked.
Finally, whenever her program came up for funding or refunding
(from at least a half-dozen or more sources), she was not content
only to describe her mode of operation and accomplishments. She
would give example after example for which she had computed the
cost of a particular resource exchange for a particular client, and
how it differed from what the cost would have been if those clients
had been served in conventional agency ways. Daphne Krause
understood and employed cost-benefit analysis. She was a born
accountant. Her grant applications were unique documents.

Daphne Krause did not seek to interconnect, to network, the
different agencies with which she dealt. There was no network to

bring them together. But in relation to each agency, she played Mrs. Dewar's coordinator role, and she did it in textbook fashion, except that there is no textbook! Her success illustrates what can be achieved between formal organizations when someone like her is on the scene, whether or not a network like ours is in operation. The similarities in results obtained by Daphne Krause and Mrs. Dewar lend force to our attempt to describe intellectual, cognitive, and personal characteristics of such coordinating people.

Key Elements of the Role

In what follows, the reader should not assume that we are completely secure about having identified all of the features of the role, or that those we have identified are as unitary as they may seem. We have no doubt about the importance of these features. We offer this caveat, obviously, because the number of coordinators with whom we have worked or supervised is not large.

Knowing the Territory

The most obvious characteristic of the coordinator is knowledge of a wide variety of individuals, agencies, and organizations in his or her arena of interest, an arena which may or may not be geographically circumscribed. By *knowledge* we do not mean mere awareness of their existence, but specific knowledge, however gained, of their resources, purposes, needs, programs, and even history. The person will usually know someone in some of the organizations or know somebody who knows someone in them. It is not knowledge passively obtained but rather a consequence of a curiosity, a seeking, that is second nature to the person. It is not curiosity about everything in a person's world, but in regard to the person's work interests. It is not a directory-style amassing of information; it is information organized in terms of people's and organizations' purposes, programs, styles, and outlooks. Depending on what you want to know, this person can suggest whom you should contact, what to expect, what resources they have, what their needs are, and how those needs may fit in with yours. We are describing a person who is likely to say, and sincerely so, "Let me know what goes. If so-and-so can't help, please get back to me and I'll see what I can come up with." In brief, by word and manner the person conveys ongoing availability and desire to stay in touch. Clearly, we are describing a combination of cognitive and personal-social characteristics that not everyone possesses, of course, and one that appears in very different degrees among those who possess it at all. People approach the subject with varying conceptual explicitness. That is, they may not label what they do and why, but they do what they do with what they know because that is the kind of person they are. How they came to be what they are can also vary considerably. A Mrs. Dewar or Daphne Krause can tell you at length how they came to think and act as they do, but there are others like them who have never felt the need to plumb and organize their pasts to understand why they think and act as they do. As we shall see later, the process by which we have interviewed and selected individuals who say they want to be coordinators is one in which some of these individuals begin to put their experiences together in ways they never had before. It is also a process that can make clear to some that whatever their virtues, capabilities, and motivations, they are not suited for a coordinating role based on a resource exchange rationale.

Scanning, Fluidity, and Imaginativeness

If anything is truly distinctive about the Mrs. Dewars and Daphne Krauses of this world, it is the ability to see mutually enhancing connections among individuals, programs, and agencies that on the surface appear to be in different worlds. Where most people see discreteness, they may see commonalities of needs, of matches or exchanges of resources. It is not only that they are scanners of their ecology, but they know the territory. More than a few people know it, but their scanning is not informed and powered by a resource exchange rationale: Who has what? Who needs what? Is there a basis for a productive exploitation of each other's strengths? They do not see individuals and organizations in terms of their conventional labels but rather in terms of what they have learned about what they do, how they do it, and what they cannot but wish to do—or do far less than they wish to do—because of a conventional view that makes resources more limited than they need be.

We have used the words *scanning*, *fluidity*, and *imaginativeness*. They are not easy to define, and dictionary definitions are not so helpful for our purposes. Everybody *scans*, but not everybody does it so as to be able to see (to want to see) underlying commonalities among surface differences. We use *fluidity* to describe both the speed and ease with which people perceive commonalities; some people arrive at those perceptions slowly; some with a speed and ease that is remarkable; and for some, A is A and B is B, and never the twain shall meet. With some people who are being exposed to a new arena of experience, fluidity may be next to nil, but once they get the point they take off. Some never do. In our experience, this has little or nothing to do with IQ, education, or experience in previous arenas. For our purposes, why this is so is less important than that this range of individual differences exists. *Imaginativeness* is the most troublesome of the three words because it too frequently is viewed as a characteristic you do or do not have in general, which we do not think to be the case. We use the word, despite its vagueness, because it gets at one of the motivating forces of scanning, i.e., a need or desire to see underlying connections or possibilities between observables that others do not see but that give you kicks. What we here call imaginativeness is both process and force.

In using such words, we are not suggesting that in combination they are a general characteristic of the person, although that is sometimes the case. Very often, the characteristic is displayed in a circumscribed arena or domain of activity and is not displayed elsewhere. Of course, it is not a "you have it or you do not have it" characteristic. But if people possess it in differing degrees, it is, to an undetermined extent, learnable. For example, in the word game

Scrabble, the player has a certain number of tiles each of which has a letter of the alphabet, some letters having a greater numerical value than others. The player starting the game seeks to use some or all of his or her tiles to form a word on the board. Whoever is next then must form a word that in some way builds upon a letter in the word of the starter—it must connect with what is on the board. There are procedural rules we need not go into here; suffice it to say that what is required is that you "allow" yourself to see possibilities for forming words, and do it in ways that capitalize on the different numerical values of your tiles. When two people play, it is not unusual for a game to take two or more hours, during which time you have truly "worked." It is a challenging game. We mention the example for two reasons. First, becoming a good Scrabble player has little to do with the extent of your vocabulary. At least among highly educated, professional people the correlation between vocabulary and articulateness, on the one hand, and adeptness in playing Scrabble on the other is not much above zero. Indeed, the variation among them can be considerable, and cause for humorous comment. Some can see possibilities and connections with what appears to be the speed of light; others seem to miss the obvious. Over time some people catch on, and others hardly improve. Strength of motivation is by no means an unimportant factor, but wanting to become a good player is not enough. The second reason we use Scrabble as an example is that the cognitive characteristics a player displays may or may not be seen in other arenas of cognitive activity.

Who can become a good Scrabble player? That is the sort of question our description of a particular kind of coordinator raises. In regard to Scrabble, the question is not answerable until the person begins to learn the game. But in regard to the coordinator, we *know* there are people who possess and employ the characteristics of scanning, fluidity, and imaginativeness (albeit in varying degrees) so highly possessed by a Mrs. Dewar or a Daphne Krause. Locating and interviewing them, and determining whether they possess other characteristics relevant to the role, are difficult issues we shall take up later.

Let us bring the issues to life with a concrete example. Dr. George Albee is a renowned psychologist, whose corpus of influential writings contains little about resource exchange or coordination except for one paper about his experience in raising and feeding pigs! Because that publication will not be available to most readers, and because the paper manages to be both instructive and entertaining (an unusual combination), we offer a long excerpt to reveal Dr. Albee's thinking about a very practical problem.[1]

> When our neighbors gave us our first pig, we began feeding it the conventional pig food (lots of corn, dry whey, and middlings) obtained in 100-pound bags at the grain store. Marge became a family pet. Even at 650 pounds she would come scampering like a puppy to have her back scratched. She bore a litter of piglets twice a year. (Each little one sells for $30, so a litter is worth $240 to $360.) A pig will grow very fast on grain. Five or six sacks will bring it to slaughter weight (180 to 200 pounds) in five or six months, with reasonable economy and efficiency. But once one observes the gusto with which a pig devours table scraps and vegetable scrapings, once one sees the relish with which a pig drinks sour milk, eats moldy cottage cheese, devours weeds pulled from the garden, gulps blemished fruits, soft tomatoes, leftover party dips, one suddenly becomes aware of the perfect match between the mountainous quantity of food that is wasted in America and the omnivorous and efficient digestive system of the pig.
>
> It became a game to see how many sources of free or inexpensive food we could find. Someone tipped us off about the availability of outdated dairy products. Every container of milk, cottage cheese, sour cream, and yogurt in the cold case at the supermarket carries a date. In most states, the dairy product may not be sold for human use after the date stamped on the carton. Dairy companies supplying the supermarkets give credit for these outdated packages

carried back to the dairy company's loading platform. Very large quantities are simply thrown away. We learned, however, that a local dairy allowed "pig men" bringing their own containers to empty the cartons and packages for a very modest charge. I discovered that I could carry away a forty-quart milk can filled to the brim with milk (or cream and other dairy products) for the nominal sum of one dollar. We quickly bought a couple more weanling piglets.

Exploring further, I learned that cheese factories have available for the asking enormous quantities of whey, a liquid rich in protein and minerals. In most states whey may not be dumped into the nearest stream or river because the lightly nutritious substance promotes the growth of algae and other plants that have a devastating polluting effect. So cheese factories give this by-product away. They practically beg people to take it. If your needs are sufficiently large, the cheese companies will even haul it to your farm in tank trucks. An enormous amount of research on the conversion of whey into animal feed is going on in agricultural colleges throughout the country. The University of Vermont's dairy gives whey to the cows instead of water. Pigs and chickens love it. The only real disadvantage of whey is that it spoils in a few days, depending on the temperature, and so it must be picked up frequently.

Other sources of free or cheap animal food kept appearing. One of my children was on a Little League baseball team last summer. His team manager happened to be in charge of the fruit and vegetable section of a large local supermarket. After some friendly conversation I arranged to pick up, late each afternoon, the day's trimmings and cullings. It was after a few days of this that we decided to buy a secondhand pickup truck!

Each day we would bring home eight to ten large boxes of deep-green lettuce and crisp cabbage leaves, quantities of bruised and overripe fruit, often whole boxes of grapes, plums, and cherries that had developed molds and mildews. Some days there would be more than a hundred pounds of overripe bananas. Root vegetables with modest defects, eggplants that were off-color, and, for some reason, enormous numbers of celery stalks found their way into our boxes.

We learned that the remarkable size and color uniformity of fruits and vegetables in the modern American supermarket is not a chance phenomenon. Sometimes we would watch as the manager and his assistants ruthlessly trimmed away the most nutritious outer leaves of head lettuce to bring all the heads to a uniform size so that they could be sold at a uniform price. Romaine, escarole, endive, chicory—the most nutritious outer leaves were trimmed off. Odd-shaped or odd-color fruits went into the reject bin. Understandably, this high rate of waste results in higher prices for the fruits and vegetables that survive.

At about this time we began sharing our incredible bounty with a neighbor who held many of our attitudes and who was experimenting with raising rabbits and geese for food. (A prolific doe rabbit, who can have a litter about every thirty days, can produce several hundred pounds of protein each year.) Rabbit is fine lean meat, delicious and nutritious. Goose is fine fat meat, delicious and nutritious.

We really began to get fascinated, and increasingly appalled, by the amount of food wasted, thrown away, ground down disposals, trucked to landfills, left to rot. One weekend, a visiting Israeli student accompanied me on my rounds of food collection for our animals. She was shocked and then indignant at American wastefulness. It happened that on that particular weekend we fell heir to an especially large quantity of ripe bananas, which our six pigs devoured with lip-smacking gusto. She estimated that her whole kibbutz could live for a week on that day's truckload of fruits and vegetables.

My wife teaches at a small liberal-arts college. One day I joined her for lunch in the college cafeteria. I became fascinated with the eating habits of undergraduates. Apparently, many show their sophistication and worldliness by tasting and rejecting as inedible or unappealing a wide variety of perfectly nutritious food. I returned a couple of times to watch the system of emptying trays, then grinding up and flushing away the enormous quantities of food left on the students' plates after each meal.

After a couple of friendly cups of coffee with the dining-hall manager I learned, too, that his cooks often threw away quantities of uneaten food. While he is fairly skilled at estimating the quantities of food ordinarily required, it is important to always plan to "have enough." There is no wrath like the wrath of the college student who is "paying good money" for room and board and who comes to dinner to find the steam table empty of one of the three entrees of the day. But unexpected events affected the eating habits of students. A rainy day may keep them in the dorms. A sunny spring day may send them into the hills, to drink in the joys of nature and to skip dinner. The leftover food goes down the giant disposal. We added the college cafeteria to our sources and decided to begin breeding piglets for sale as well as for family use.

But the greatest food bonanza was yet to come. One evening after a buffet dinner at our house for a group of graduate students, I was following my usual procedure of scraping the plates into the chicken bucket. A graduate student who had stayed on to help clean up revealed that she worked part-time, evenings and weekends, at a local motel restaurant. One of the chefs, a man in his late twenties, was a concerned environmentalist. She brought us together. He had started as a busboy ten years before and was now the head evening chef for an excellent, successful, and very busy restaurant and lunch counter in the motel. The motel also has large banquet facilities, and the efficient kitchen was responsible for several banquets each week, serving from fifty to four hundred people. He agreed with my comments and expanded on his experience with the wasteful food habits of Americans. After some discussion and exploration we worked out an agreement where I would pay the motel $20 a month, provide clean galvanized garbage cans each day, and make a daily pickup of the enormous quantities of leftover food that had been flushed down the restaurant disposal for years. Shortly thereafter I worked out an arrangement with another farm family to pick up the animal diet on alternate days, because the quantity was more than our small pig operation could consume. We also decided to build a modest 14-by-30-foot pole barn.

Once one's consciousness is raised in the matter of food waste, one begins to observe the phenomenon everywhere. For a time my children had to pull me back from prowling behind the counters of pizza palaces, poking in to the trash barrels at McDonald's, and wandering down alleys back of restaurants. I became the despair of my trash-collection company, a local free-enterprise operation. Twice the company raised my weekly fee because of the quantity of boxes, fruit crates, and dairy containers that we piled up for it each week. With a sudden flash of awareness, I realized that the driver must be taking the trash somewhere and that with my truck I could do the same thing. I discovered a world that few upper-middle-class Americans encounter: the town dump (more frequently referred to as the sanitary landfill). Trash is dumped in an area adjacent to a mountain largely composed of sand, so that huge bulldozers can engage in the never-ending task of covering over the rejected material and debris of a wasteful industrial civilization. I found the town dump, and the men who work there, a great further source of information on our wasteful culture. I also discovered that the town dump is a great source of all sorts of items useful to a part-time farmer with some serendipity [Albee, 1977, pp. 65–67].

It is fascinating that once Dr. Albee grasped the matching principle he was off and running. He became a seeker of matches, some of which clearly involved resource exchange. From what he wrote, it is as if he found a new game that had practical payoff and at the same time was intellectual fun, especially because the places he located for his needs were, on the surface, wildly different from each other.

Would Dr. Albee make a good coordinator? That he possesses the characteristics of scanning, fluidity, and imaginativeness in regard to food for his pigs does not necessarily mean that he would have those characteristics in regard to people, agencies, and other formal organizations. (Because we know Dr. Albee and his professional organizational accomplishments, we feel secure in saying he would make a good coordinator.)

Perceiving Assets and Building on Strengths

It is, in our opinion, no exaggeration to assert that most people are disposed to be more aware of the deficits of others than of their assets. This is especially true for medical and human services personnel, whose training almost guarantees such a mind-set, but it is only slightly less the case for people in other kinds of formal organization. The consequences are several. First, it concentrates resources for the purpose of repair; prevention goes by the board. Second, the perception and use of assets (individual, organizational) tend not to be central to the picture—when they are in the picture at all. Third, the concentration on deficits tends to be acontextual, i.e., the single individual or agency is not seen in relation to other individuals or agencies that conceivably could be interconnected in mutually productive ways. Fourth, the concentration, in practice, has the effect of increasing the number of individuals and agencies who are perceived as having certain deficits, thereby requiring that more resources be used to train more people to deal with those deficits; also, in practice, the concentration tends to increase the number of specialists needed for the repair effort.[2]

We are not saying that deficits are not real. By a near-exclusive concentration on them, you and the object of your helping efforts place emphasis on what someone lacks or cannot do, and you downplay what an individual has and can do, i.e., you start with deficits (the emphasis on pathology) and you increase awareness of them, too often ignoring possibilities for building on existing assets.

"Perceiving assets and building on strengths." For some people, the words have the ring of Pollyanna-ish virtue: high-sounding, noble, head-in-the-clouds words that fly in the face of reality. But the real world provides instance after instance of the practical consequences of taking assets seriously: not ignoring lacks but essentially redefining them so that what one party lacks becomes an asset to someone else, and vice versa. For example, Dr. Richard Sussman once found himself helping a school district cope with the problem of keeping bright, college-bound seniors from goofing off in their final semester. He also knew a professor of child development who was very keen to do research in local elementary schools but had been unable to gain access to them. With some initial difficulty, he persuaded the professor to have her graduate students train high school students to collect, organize, and analyze data for her research, in return for permission for the high school students to employ their new skills on her research questions in the district's elementary schools. The project satisfied the needs of both parties very well, and the participating high school students even gave presentations at the sponsoring university and to their own board of education. No money ever changed hands, but both sides were far richer as a result of the collaboration.

It was also Dr. Sussman who once set up a housing exchange among the clients of two service agencies. One was trying to find shelter for homeless women with children, and for young married couples. The other was trying to help seniors stay in their homes, despite increasing needs for care and help around the house. With careful attention to the personalities and capabilities on both sides, he was able to match over twenty sets of people, exchanging company and care for shelter. Most of the matches were successful, and not one led to dangerous consequences. Nonetheless, though both agencies appreciated the value of the demonstration, neither felt able to assign a staff member to the project, which was allowed to lapse after Dr. Sussman left it.

In the organizational world, the mind-set to perceive assets and build on strengths is infrequently found. However, it is our experience that there are individuals to whom the mind-set is congenial so that once they grasp it, they respond with an "of course." We have to add from personal experience, though, that it becomes a cognitive characteristic of a person only after a struggle. For some the struggle is not long, for others it is, and for still others it never becomes second nature. Determining whether a person already has (to some degree) that mind-set, or has the ability to acquire it, is a problem for which we now have no clear answer. We return to the point later in this chapter.

Power, Influence, and Selflessness

The type of coordinator we are attempting to describe has no formal power. He or she is a suggester, a source of possibilities, a convener, an acquirer of knowledge about the purposes and needs of individuals, organizations, and their parts. By words and style of action, the coordinator conveys a clear message:

> I have no power to direct or mandate. I do not represent a tribunal of judgment. My sole task is to come up with, to suggest, possible ways your purposes and needs can be met by interconnecting with others with whom you now have no interconnections; all suggestions need agreement from both sides in order to proceed. You are free to pursue or reject the possibilities I suggest. If you wish to pursue them, you can count on my availability to be of whatever help I can be. I will not criticize what you are doing or not doing, nor do I control any resources I can assign to you, but in light of the needs you have, I will try to come up with ways for those needs to be met, to some degree at least. What I come up with may sometimes strike you as unconventional, or impractical, or off the wall. All I ask is that you think about it and let me know what you come up with.

This message cannot be conveyed by someone who has a strong need to direct, mandate, or control—which immediately rules out a lot of people. The coordinator might have such a need, fantasy, or ambition, but it is controlled by the knowledge and belief that *requiring* people to change their accustomed ways of thinking and working is frequently—some will say almost always—counterproductive. The literature on organizations is replete with examples where the commandment "Thou shalt coordinate" creates far more problems than it resolves. To offer a point that bears repeating, when we emphasize that this role is without formal power, it is not because we think power is inherently sinful and to be avoided at all costs at all times; rather, for the purposes of the role, in our experience possessing power is almost always self-defeating.

Not having power does not mean, of course, being without influence. How much influence the coordinator comes to have depends largely, as it always does, on personal style and ideas. Books have been written about the origins and development of a style or personality. Suffice it to say here that the role we are describing calls for a person who is likeable, outgoing but not pushy, tactful, inquiring but not intrusive, a listener—someone who has the patience to let people ponder a suggestion for days before calling them to follow up on the meeting, and someone who can help people think without making them feel they are being forced to do or think anything.

It would appear that we are describing a paragon of virtue, a secular angel. The fact is that there are such people. Their number is not large, but as we shall see shortly, it may be larger than we think. We must hasten to add that in our limited experience in selecting, supervising, or advising coordinators none of them had all the listed characteristics to the same degree. Indeed, some of them lacked this or that characteristic to a degree that could be troublesome, i.e., they could be impatient, too directive, or too easily subject to feelings of rejection when their suggestions produced no action. We should also add that in initially meeting these individuals we felt they appeared to be markedly different from each other; the characteristics they shared were not initially apparent.

A Parallel Position

In building up a picture of the ideal coordinator, it may be useful to consider the work of Dr. Alan Towbin in a very different field. His approach to the work of psychoanalysis—a term he now rejects— has much the same impact as that of Mrs. Dewar on organizational collaboration. Here he speaks for himself:[3]

> I used to be a psychotherapist and some people would insist that I am one still. How, then, did I come to think of myself as a professional confidant, engaging clients in a confiding relationship? For a

long time I had been in intellectual agreement with Szasz that the concept of mental illness is a myth, an arbitrary way of responding to the behavior of troubled and troubling people. Oh, I could see how this model of behavior and the healing relationship it supported could be and indeed often were used oppressively. But my agreement with Szasz remained a conviction without force until I experienced my own professional activity in the mental illness system—being a healer—as being party to the system's oppression of its clients. At that point my commitments to the principle "don't make things worse" and to my role as a healer became incompatible. I went through a period of crisis and quit my job in an institutional setting. But that didn't settle the ethical issue. Even in private practice I had "patients," did "treatment," and engaged in the lucrative rituals of the healing relationship: made diagnoses and signed forms for clients whose insurance "covered" mental illness. Convinced that the role of healer was a dishonest and oppressive way of relating to people I didn't believe were ill, there was nothing to do but abandon it. In its place I gradually developed the conception of my work as that of a professional confidant.

It was easy enough to tell my clients that they were not getting a healer, that I offered no treatment, did not regard them as "sick," would make no diagnoses, and kept no case records. Finding a positive way of portraying the relationship was harder. With little reflection I spoke of myself as "like a confidant—someone you feel you can talk to about anything, without having to worry that it might damage your relationship. Well, I'm a professional confidant." Over a period of five years, a series of several hundred clients accepted this definition of our relationship and replied to my inquiry that they had no currently functional confidant [1978, p. 333].*

---

*It should be noted that Elizabeth Lorentz does not view Towbin's paper as relevant to or consistent with the rationale central to this book, on the grounds that his thinking is embedded in a helper-helpee tradition that is antithetical to the role of a coordinator as

Central to Towbin's position is the proposition that "the ordinary, naturally occurring relation between confider and confidant in everyday life is the model for the client-professional relationship in practice" (p. 336). So what does he do with and say to a client? He tries to "be the best confidant for this confider" (p. 336) that he can—with no set agenda to follow, simply staying in the moment and paying full attention to the client. He continues:

> The "purposelessness" of the professional confidant's activity seems to pose the most difficult problem in characterizing the relationship. Because the model in the confiding-relationship paradigm refers to a relation that occurs naturally and is informal, we would not expect to find a task orientation in the confidant. But for a professional our expectations are different. There we expect to meet an expert who conducts an enterprise. In western culture, enterprise has a (paradigmatic) form, without which the activity appears meaningless. Thus, the task must be approached planfully, the necessary tools and materials collected, the former applied to the latter with skill, and an anticipated result is, or perhaps is not, achieved. There is a beginning, a middle, and an end. Although our cultural training leads us to see *this* form as natural or inevitable, and its absence as chaos, perhaps we can still appreciate that this reaction is itself *paradigmatic*. Contemporary artists have abandoned this concept of form, and their works do often elicit strong negative emotion from people trained in the traditional aesthetic. The confiding relationship paradigm posits a similarly "formless" relation within the structure of the contract. Like the natural confiding relationship, *the relationship the professional offers is not a means for getting somewhere or producing an effect: it stands only for itself!* [pp. 336–337; italics are Towbin's].

---

we have described it. Sarason agrees in part but is impressed with the process of resource definition that allowed Towbin to see himself and his clients in a new light. We leave it to the reader to make his or her own judgment. The disagreement between the authors was real. We tossed a coin and Sarason won.

In this view, clients are simply ordinary people who are upset and in need of someone to confide in. The best response is thus to be a good confidant—not a detached professional with special healing powers, but someone solidly centered in personal feelings. The role requires objectivity, but of the kind that "rests on the professional confidant being a certain kind of person on the one hand, and on the absence of a task or task orientation, on the other" (p. 337).

Dr. Towbin goes on to report something truly unusual:

In my earlier attempt to conceptualize the role of the professional confidant, I noted that if we want to know what a confiding relationship is like, we have only to look about us in the world.

About a year later, I took my own advice and put the following ad in the "personals" column of the local paper:

Do people confide in you? I would like to meet with you if you have no professional background. I am a licensed psychologist. If you are interested, call 776–_____ and leave your name and number for Dr. _____.

I hoped for a dozen replies and got over 100. Of the 19 people I've seen face to face, two were openly so anxious that they distinguish themselves from the remaining 17 in this situation, although perhaps not in relations with people they know. So I'll limit myself to a characterization of these 17, thirteen women and four men.

They had highly varied backgrounds. . . . As varied as their statistics were, these people functioned in a remarkably similar way in the interview. I had met one of them socially a few months earlier, but otherwise I was a stranger to all. Yet all appeared calm and at ease when we met and all but two were spontaneously very sociable and friendly in manner; these two warmed up more slowly. All faced me directly, seemed to fix me with their gaze, made excellent eye-contact, and conveyed I had their undivided attention throughout the interview. These actions, and perhaps other behaviors of which I'm not aware, contributed to a strong impression of being with someone who is fully "present." All seemed self-possessed with an air of being on top of things. They characterized themselves as self-confident, secure in the conviction that they could handle their own lives effectively. When they spoke of their family backgrounds and relations with confiders, each of them seemed completely open in their reports, often on serious matters, deeply felt; for example, the recent or imminent death of a beloved parent. They appeared sincere and concerned in such reports; there was no emotionality or dramatization of the situation—though occasional flashes of ironic humor occurred.

These 17 people came across to me as personally appealing people, enthusiastically interested in what we were doing together, warm and candid, with marked presence and a convincing air of self-confidence and competence. As a popular expression would have it, they seemed to "have their act together." If they convey to others what I saw and felt, it's no wonder that many people seek them out as confidants.

Our interest is a particular type of coordinating role, not a therapeutic or semitherapeutic one. Nevertheless, there are aspects of Towbin's thinking and action that are similar to ours.

- *The emphasis in the relationship focuses on and emphasizes the confider's strengths rather than deficits.* Similarly, the focus of the coordinator is on what resources the person has and can apply to the matter at hand.

- *The confidant has no power, and seeks none.* He or she has no "technique"; influence is a consequence of an ability "to convey an intense, compassionate interest in the confider." Many psychotherapists now accept the premise that it is the therapist's presence as a person and not technique that is a prerequisite to effective psychotherapy. That ability is what enables a person willingly to ponder the coordinator's suggestions or possibilities for matching.

- *The confidant is available.* There are no traditional, professional time constraints on the duration of contact or the number of contacts. There is no predetermined end point.

Similarly, the coordinator's time perspective is "open" and imposes no time pressures on those with whom he or she meets. What a person brings up, and the pace with which the person accepts or rejects (in whole or in part) a possibility the coordinator suggests, is determined by the person without being associated with value judgments on the part of the coordinator. Coordinators have *influence* as much by virtue of the kind of people they are as by cognitive-intellectual characteristics or how much sheer knowledge they have.

"The confidants exemplify a mode of functioning which many experts in psychology regard as vital, *and which is a spontaneous, unschooled expression of their personalities*" (italics ours). We found precisely the same with many of those in the coordinator role we have described, a goodly number of whom had not known us at all. This brings us to Dr. Towbin's surprise and delight at the number of people who answered his ad. Without in any way suggesting that the number of people who have the *combination* of characteristics we think an effective coordinator should have is large, we now believe that the number is larger than we initially thought. As Towbin notes, "Pancoast and Collins describe a population of helpers they call 'natural neighbors' in much the same terms as I have used to describe confidants. One function natural neighbors serve is that of confidant to others. These authors cite other studies on natural helpers in 'networks,' a concept applicable to the functioning of many of the confidants described here."

There are differences between the roles of coordinator and confidant. The confidant is in a one-to-one helping relationship, whereas the coordinator aims to foster interactions among *others* in the network, i.e., relationships that affect the outlooks and activities of people in the network. *The coordinator is no confidant*. Nonetheless, Towbin's paper makes a significant and relevant point, one too often ignored: although an individual may be motivated to be in a role and may intellectually comprehend the role, it does not follow that the individual has the personal style or characteristics to do justice to the spirit and letter of the role. You may want to be a confidant like Towbin, but you may not be the kind of person who can do justice to the role. Similarly, we have known people who very much wanted to be network coordinators but who could not stay within the confines of the role, i.e., they were too directive, impatient, passive, or intrusive. As we said earlier, there are teachers who should not be teachers, doctors who should not be doctors, etc. How to locate and select network coordinators is a very thorny problem. The most able and successful coordinators are those who previously were performing *most* aspects of the role although (like Towbin's confidants) they never had need to pin the label on themselves.

In our experience, the combination of characteristics we have described in this chapter is possessed in varying degrees by some individuals in formal organizations. But such individuals are not recognized as having this asset and, given the rationale and structure of those organizations, there is no way of capitalizing on the asset. The assets are ready to be mined, but there are no miners. Our experience has been largely with and in informal resource exchange networks created so that members (singly or otherwise) could draw on a pool of resources, needs, and interests pertinent to their own. This has made it more likely that individuals would come to the fore who appeared to have the combination of characteristics a coordinator needed to have. Indeed, it would be more correct to say that they were attracted to join and remain in the network because they already had, in varying degrees, some of these necessary characteristics even though they worked in formal organizations where those characteristics were difficult to express or implement on the level of action.

Selecting Coordinators

It follows from what we have said that the important question is not how to train coordinators but whom to train for the role.

We have found there are several ways to identify effective coordinators. None of them involves "scouting" in the sense that we deliberately went looking for a potential coordinator. Because each

of the writers was involved in numerous organizations and, therefore, attended scads of meetings, we could not avoid observing and
listening to individuals who seemed to have a grasp of the resource
exchange rationale. We made it our business to get to know them,
and if they were not aware of our network, we would briefly
describe our activities. We would invite them to attend network
meetings. A fair number of them did just that and provided us the
opportunity to observe them. Seeing how they operated at our
meetings allowed us to judge whether they in fact could act in
accord with our rationale and, no less important, whether they possessed the different personal stylistic characteristics of a coordinator we discussed earlier. In some cases, if we felt the person was not
suited for the role, we said nothing about providing supervision;
that is, they remained active members of the network engaged in
resource exchanges with other members that were mutually
rewarding. In other instances where we had little doubt about the
person's suitability, Mrs. Dewar initiated a series of meetings to go
into the dilemmas and opportunities of the coordinator's role in
great depth. On the surface, the role seems a relatively simple one,
and it was Mrs. Dewar's task to point out how personally demand-
ing it can be. As examples, the coordinator suggests but does not
direct; one has to know the contexts in which people work in order
to see possibilities of resource exchange; the coordinator has much
to do *before* a network meeting takes place and follow-up is required
after the meeting; it is crucial to be available to members seeking
information and advice; one stays in touch with members without
being perceived as intrusive or directive; and the success of a network depends not on the coordinator as "leader" but as a catalyst
for enlarging members' views of their resources and those of others.

Potential coordinators were also identified as someone would
read our books, or hear of the Northern Westchester Network, and
call Mrs. Dewar to say he or she wished to become a coordinator
and seek her help. When Mrs. Dewar met with the person, she
conducted a very searching interview to determine how well the
person understood the rationale, how and with what frequency the

rationale was employed, whether the person knew community organizations and had relationships with them, and whether the person understood the time demands and obligations of the coordinator. These initial meetings ran two or more hours. If the person was within driving distance of a network meeting, he or she was invited to attend and to leave discussion of becoming a coordinator for a later time. There were several individuals who lived in other states; their subsequent discussions were held by telephone. Mrs. Dewar tried to be helpful, and we have reason to believe that in a handful of instances these telephone discussions were beneficial, if one goes by what they reported by phone or in writing.

A crucial point is that when Mrs. Dewar would agree to supervise a person, she truly supervised. The person observed and worked with her, not only seeing what she did but learning why she did it. It was an intensive one-on-one relationship.

We do not claim that the criteria we employed for selection and the quality and substance of the supervised experience cannot (or should not) be improved. We were always learning as we went along. For a variety of reasons, we were never in the position of doing what we very much wanted to do: to develop a research program by which we could attract and study a cadre of individuals desiring to become coordinators, i.e., a program that could serve as a basis for self-correction in regard to selecting and training. We had to be content (albeit very reluctantly) with description and presentation of our conceptual and action rationale. In addition to what we have described and written, Thompson's detailed and extensive study (1985) of the Northern Westchester Network is very important.

Two things seem to be essential to a potential coordinator. The first is a constructive way of thinking, i.e., the ability to avoid riveting attention on people's deficits but rather to see and build on strengths. The second is the ability to see opportunities for connections between people or organizations that appear to be entirely separate. A person can have those assets, however, and still do a miserable job of coordination.

Conclusion

We are describing a particular kind of person in a particular kind of role. It is a role that does not exist, but should, in and among formal organizations. It can be found informally, outside of organizations, albeit with varying breadth and duration and with an anonymity that has successfully prevented organizational theorists and practitioners from seeing its accomplishments for the plaguing problem of coordination.

This chapter has not done justice either to the characteristics of the coordinator or to the selection of such a person. It is not in the cards, given the lack of attention that these kinds of role and person have gotten, and given the fact that our experience has been in an admittedly narrow (and informal) context, although over a very long period of time. But the more we reflected on our experience, and the more we observed failure after failure of efforts to achieve "coordination" in and among formal organizations, we felt justified, indeed compelled, to write about what we have experienced and learned. As noted in Chapter Two, when a problem appears to be wholly or in part intractable, it is a sure sign that there is something wrong or missing in our assumptions and ways of thinking. It is also a sign that when and if what is missing or wrong is identified, resistance to its implications will be very strong and people will come up with all kinds of reasons for dismissing it. Sometimes, of course, what is identified makes little sense or is impractical, perhaps utopian, and deserves not to be taken seriously. Obviously, in regard to the role we have described, we regard such dismissal as totally unwarranted. We did not dream up the role. Our view of it stems only in small part from our subjective opinions. In our earlier books and this one, we have tried to describe in detail how and why the role is a productive one. And we hope we have made clear that one of the starting points for our endeavor was the knowledge that the "coordination problem" is seemingly intractable. We were not tilting at windmills.

Notes

1. *Country Journal*, March 1977, pp. 62–67. Reprinted with the permission of Dr. George Albee.

2. An example is the 1975 federal legislation about services for handicapped children. With each passing year, the number of children deemed eligible for services has dramatically increased—as have, of course, fiscal outlays, the number of professional specialists, and the use of time as a resource. This has taken place even though, beginning with the implementation of legislation, observers pointed out that many children were diagnosed as having certain deficits they did not in fact possess or possessed minimally and never should have been stigmatized.

   We recall a most egregious example, reported once on the front page of the *New York Times*. One of the most prestigious private schools in the country initiated a deficit-oriented diagnostic program, costing a lot of money, with the result that a large majority of students were found to possess cognitive deficits. Practically no student was "normal." Our experience with the 1975 federal legislation abundantly confirms what the article reports. We are not mindless critics of professionalism, but the reality is that one of the occupational hazards of deficit-oriented professionals is that they are too ready to see the deficits for which their training prepared them. As someone once said, "When your only tool is a hammer, every problem starts to look like a nail."

3. From Towbin (1978); reprinted with permission of Dr. Alan Towbin.

Chapter Six

Collegiality and Community

The New Paradigm in Action

Any socially complicated organization has problems and conflicts about resources, communication, collegiality, and the need to adapt to new circumstances. This is predictable, a given, a realistic expectation. But when these conflicts and problems persist and are intractable to efforts to lessen their negative consequences, it is most unlikely that the organization will survive.

In this context, it is useful to consider what happened to the American private sector in the post–World War II era. For more than three decades after the war, the private sector operated on the assumption that the future would be a carbon copy of the past and present, i.e., what had worked to make American business the world's business giant ensured its continued dominance. It didn't work out that way. Germany, and especially Japan, made dramatic inroads on that dominance, and there came a time when it not only seemed many American companies would go under but the country's monetary and fiscal stability required it to be dependent on foreign investments and the purchase of government securities. The American automotive industry was a clear example of what was happening, but by no means the only one.

How to explain this? What permitted Japanese and German business and industry to be so successful? A new generation of CEOs, organizational theorists, and researchers began to provide answers. Essentially, they indicted a smug, insensitive, unimaginative style of leadership that defined human resources in the narrowest of ways, resisted change, confused organization charts with organizational realities, and also confused mandated coordination with achieved coordination. That leadership pronounced anathema on boundary crossing within the organization, as well as on seeking to exchange knowledge and resources with other companies, even though those exchanges could be mutually rewarding.

Meanwhile, at the same time that much of American business and industry was on a downhill course, some companies were taking the themes that we outline in this book seriously and with ever-increasing success. They knew that they had to change; the traditional rationale undergirding organizational structure was self-defeating; the definition, garnering, coordination, and exchange of resources within and among companies were both necessary and productive; and the forging and nurturing of networks discernibly increased collegiality, community, and the size of the bottom line. Wonder of wonders, these companies, many of which sought global markets and connections, quickly learned that their first tasks were to understand foreign settings and companies in terms of their distinctive cultures and to adopt strategies that took such understanding seriously.

Collaborative Advantage

Over a period of three years, Rosabeth Kanter and her research group studied thirty-seven companies and their partnerships, concentrating on international and cross-cultural relationships among them. She coined the phrase *collaborative advantage* to describe the benefit companies can derive from such partnerships—a phrase that organizations of all types would do well to keep in mind: "In the global economy, a well-developed ability to create and sustain fruitful collaborations gives companies a significant competitive leg up" (1994, p. 96). At the same time, she observed that many companies missed out on much of the potential benefit because top management "worry more about controlling the relationship than about nurturing it." (See Kanter, 1995, for a more detailed analysis of the work described here.)

Kanter gives example after example, on the basis of which she outlines three essential features of productive business alliances.

They must be open-ended, yielding both immediate benefits and long-term opportunities that cannot be foreseen at the time the parties enter into the relationship. They must go beyond simple exchange of value for value to true *collaboration*, where the parties create new value together that neither of them can establish on its own. And—most important from our point of view—"They cannot be 'controlled' by formal systems but require a dense web of interpersonal connections and internal infrastructures that enhance learning" (1994, p. 97). Ideally, an intercompany agreement begins with a specific project for the partners to undertake at once—something that will give their people practice at working together and let them begin to measure the performance of the relationship. It is a poor idea to launch a partnership without doing anything concrete, she warns; "The longer a courtship drags on without consummation, the more likely conditions or minds or both can change and jeopardize it" (p. 103).

Kanter is no knee-jerk, conventional organizational theorist and practitioner, let alone someone with an antibusiness bias. She certainly is no utopian, although we do not regard it as coincidental that early in her career she wrote about utopian communities in which productively living and working together depended on some of the same factors she describes today (Kanter, 1972). At the same time, she is very clear as to the implications of her observations for conventional thinking about formal organizations. She points out that conventional Western companies tend to assume that the best managers are professionals working under specific and limited contracts, and that a professional manager can manage any corporation. This "rational" model of business management, she observes, is generally regarded as the ultimate form of organization. Unfortunately, this model does not serve well in the face of intercompany relationships, which require a "more familylike and less rational" approach: "The best intercompany relationships are frequently messy and emotional, involving feelings like chemistry or trust" (1994, p. 100).

What is most refreshing to us is Kanter's assertion that coordination is not something legislated by fiat from on high, accompanied by rhetoric about the virtues of coordination and efficiency, and based on the truly utopian assumption that language leads to actions consistent with intent. Kanter makes clear what practically everyone tends to ignore: collaboration involves *unlearning and learning*. The kind of collaboration that Kanter and we talk about is a challenge to conventional thinking; it requires changing one's accustomed way of viewing one's working role, style, and purposes.

For active, productive collaboration to take place, Kanter asserts, the organizations need a lot of contact points. Many individuals at many different levels in each organization must be involved to ensure that both partners' resources are appropriately engaged and both partners' needs and goals are met. "Broad synergies born on paper do not develop in practice until many people in both organizations know one another personally and become willing to make the effort to exchange technology, refer clients, or participate on joint teams." This involvement specifically must include the top executives of each organization, both at the beginning and on an ongoing basis; if they abandon the relationship to others in their organizations, they will lose out on opportunities to solve problems and capitalize on the partnership. At the same time, the companies should establish "formal integrator roles," assigning to some individuals the specific duty of watching for and taking advantage of opportunities for tactical integration.

Kanter's work illuminates facets of intergroup coordination ordinarily glossed over, and this is in the private sector, where our direct experience has been limited. Also, she describes a role that requires individuals to have a combination of conceptual and personal characteristics, not just one individual but multiple people at different levels and places in organizations; further, she offers the hypothesis that explicitly recognizing and creating such a role is vital to achieving the goals of what she calls collaboration and what we call coordination. Furthermore, she does not shrink from saying that she is describing a role and processes that can seem messy to those who are devotees of the precision that organization charts convey—a messiness whose consequences can be unpredictably productive, in contrast to a deceptive precision that in reality is an obstacle to new ideas, possibilities, boundary crossing, productive growth, and the sense of unlearning, learning, and personal growth. Kanter is no mindless advocate of "togetherness," as if good will (like love) is enough. Her argument is incomprehensible unless one sees it as a critique of or reaction to conventional, problem-producing conceptions of how formal organizations should look. Our own *indirect* experience with private-sector organizations confirms Kanter's observation that in the United States the conventional view is by far the predominant one. If anything, our experience suggests that the situation is worse in the public sector than in the private sector.

Kanter makes it clear that for the collaborative process to percolate within and between organizations, the top executives must gain an understanding and develop a rationale for the process, i.e., they have to become models for others, they have to understand that the rationale is not absorbed by osmosis or contagion. But how should this be accomplished? How do you select people at those multiple levels? Are not some people more appropriate than others? How can people can be aided to think and act differently in ways consistent with the collaborative rationale? What mechanisms or forums might exist that would support these people in changing to a role that is new and messy? What alterations in power relationships and status have to occur? Kanter suggests "establishing formal integrator roles." What are the *predictable* problems creating such a role would engender, and how does one prevent or dilute the untoward consequences of those problems? Does "formal" come with the *power* to integrate, in contrast to the responsibility to suggest, to articulate, *possibilities for collaboration*? How does one decide this on a basis that does not subvert the potential of the role for discerning possibilities for productive coordination?

Kanter's article (1994) understandably does not contain detailed descriptions of cases that permit us to answer the what, when, who, and why questions, varying as the answers must in light of Kanter's statement that the companies differed in their understanding of and commitment to collaboration. This is the point: if there is anything we can count on, it is that people will dramatically differ in how they think about the collaborative-coordinating rationale, its implications and implementations, and the organizational and personal changes it may require. The differences will be found within and among collaborative organizations.

Kanter's emphasis, based on her observational research, is on the rationale for collaboration, a rationale similar to ours. Our emphasis is on the cognitive *and* personal characteristics of those who will be in a particular kind of collaborative-coordinating role. Who is in that role, how well the person understands the rationale, his or her cognitive-personal characteristics, and the place and scope of the role are crucial factors that cannot be oversimplified, let alone ignored. Our experience leaves no doubt that assenting to the rationale is far easier than grasping its significance to a degree that does not allow you to view the role as you would a conventional one. It is an unconventional role that requires unconventional people, in a context seeking to depart from the conventional way of thinking and doing business.

We hope that Kanter's work stimulates discussion. At the very least, she is one of the few who have avoided contributing to pious, empty rhetoric about the coordinating role. Put more positively, she has identified one of the most egregious blind spots in organizational theory and our contemporary world. She has demonstrated that the productive use of an organization's resources depends less on its formal properties and technological sophistication than it does on its ability to define and redefine who and what is a resource and the protean ways people, purposes, and things can be viewed.

Flexible Networks

Now let us turn to the Appalachian Center for Economic Networks (ACEnet), situated in a poor, rural section of Ohio.[1] ACEnet takes on the sort of intergroup coordinating role we recommend, with a view to helping low-income individuals establish businesses or find employment in new or expanding businesses. The center's current projects involve what it calls *flexible manufacturing networks*, which "bring together groups of small firms to collaboratively manufacture items for custom or niche markets that they can't produce by themselves." One network develops home-accessibility products, another specialty food products.

The group's purposes are far from modest. To enable unemployed and low-income underemployed people to work for or own businesses, to revitalize a regional economy, to foster collaboration among small firms, to create new products and markets, to provide ongoing research and writing on the work in progress—and to do these things as a way of transforming relationships in communities and regions—is remarkable.

The ACEnet report (Holley & Borgstrom, n.d.) contrasts the usual community-action projects—born amid high hopes, only to die within a few years for lack of resources or opportunity to use their products—with its own approach of linking up such projects with local businesses. In its specialty food project, for example, it helped an association of small-scale producers identify high-value markets for processed food and apply lessons from similar associations in northern Italy (as described in Lipnack and Stamps, 1993). As the report points out:

> Increasingly, ACEnet takes on the role of the facilitator of new projects. It convenes a group composed of community-based organizations, schools, and human service agencies to develop a microenterprise program so that people on public assistance can start their own food processing firms. The local technical college opens their culinary arts kitchen to microentrepreneurs to use on nights and weekends to try out their products and their business. Volunteers from the local religious community begin to meet with some of the microentrepreneurs to design a system of support for the people transitioning from welfare that includes strategies for emergency child care and transportation.

The process spread rapidly through the community ACEnet serves. ACEnet helped a low-income advocacy group that was providing cooking classes for its membership (while encouraging them to explore microenterprise programs) to make arrangements with a county Meals on Wheels production facility to develop the latter as a training site for the former. "Presently," the report continues,

> several of the nonprofits . . . actively encourage their staff to social-ize together on Friday afternoons at a local restaurant. The number of new projects in the community have begun to multiply rapidly, springing from an increasingly dense network of relationships built up as staff from organizations in the area communicate more fre-quently with each other through formal and informal channels. Weaving these activities together is encouraged as several of the nonprofits build their skills in framing the activities under the rubric of complex concepts such as "Rural Regeneration" and sustainable development.

Several things are clear. First, ACEnet's rationale is not about individual firms, or groups, or agencies; nor is it about communities or regions, but rather about their *interdependence*—which, if not taken seriously, puts limitations on everyone's aspirations. Second, the emphasis is not on the deficits or frailties of firms, groups, indi-viduals, and agencies, but on their assets, i.e., the existing strengths on which one can build. Third, to build on such strengths requires not only a redefinition process but a variety of means that make collaboration—the recognition of practical resource exchange—a viable alternative to past practices. Fourth, when collaboration takes hold, possibilities previously not considered come to the fore, usually increasing the number and variety of participants. Fifth, sus-taining collaboration is also a process of community participation and education.

The key to the ACEnet approach is recognition that its partic-ipants' world is made up of complex systems of systems rather than of individuals and simple, unitary organizations able to act on their own without concern for each other. Survival in a world of systems requires continuous adaptation, and ACEnet has developed a niche for itself as a specialist in change dynamics, helping people "look for complex connections that begin to create a sustainable community." To cite one vivid example from the report:

When people are encouraged to see linkages, they tend to organize single activities or projects in ways that have a much wider impact on their community. For example, when people in a community decide to develop a woodlot management program, they are encouraged to work with schools so that customized training programs can be designed and institutionalized, and thus [are] more likely to last. Are woodlot owners encouraged to link with small manufacturers so that the process of making wood into final product can generate additional income for the community? Are those manufacturers getting assistance in identifying high-value products? Are low-income people having opportunities to gain jobs created by this business expansion? What resources are available to help sawmills modernize? Can new businesses be created that utilize sawdust as a raw material?

For people to understand that every action within their community has meaning, and that it can help build sustainability in many ways, is crucial. When woodlot owners work closely with small area manufacturers instead of exporting logs, they have a greater chance of creating more jobs in the community, which has many direct and indirect benefits for both groups and . . . the community as a whole.

Sustainable development is another key concept. ACEnet helps its participants add value to their products both in terms of material production and community organization, linking all areas of the community, from education and religion to banking and manufacturing, so as to "build a more healthy and equitable society." Sustainable activities, the report points out, must locate the immediate work at hand within the larger context of the community. Analyzing this goal, the report comes up with as clear a statement of our position as we have ever seen: "Staff of local organizations need to understand how crucial it is that reframing become woven throughout each interaction with others in the community, often through the use of simple questions: 'Who else should we get involved in this project? How can this project open more opportunities for people with low incomes? How will this affect our resource base?'"

Although we were naturally delighted with that statement, we could not help wondering whether it represented a pious hope or a real procedure for catalyzing productive collaborations among private-sector firms, individual entrepreneurs, and a variety of public, nonprofit community groups. The sentiment is excellent, but the report tells little or nothing about how this was done, how the inevitable problems were encountered and overcome, and who the key people were. Rationales are crucial starting points, but they require individuals to implement them in ways consistent with the rationales. Who were these individuals and what are their characteristics?

We met with ACEnet's president, June Holley, for several hours, and we have talked on the telephone for several more. Those probing (perhaps intrusively so) talks convinced us that what she and her coauthor too briefly described in their paper was probably largely valid, and that projects in the works stood an excellent chance of succeeding.

What is June Holley like? The most succinct answer is that she possesses abundantly every characteristic of the coordinator we discussed in Chapter Five. She knows the territory, she sees possibilities for matches when others do not, she is the opposite of doctrinaire or directive, she has influence but does not seek power, and she has what may best be called "community street smarts." She describes ACEnet as an "intermediary organization." June Holley is the kind of intermediary "coordinator" we have been advocating for and trying to describe—and she has been able to bring her abilities to bear on the problem of melding the public and private sectors.

It is interesting to note that the ACEnet report does more than conceptualize the interdependence of communities and regions. It takes the next, necessary step to show how and why interdependence must not ignore national and global economic transformations that can or will have an impact on local communities and regions. There are more than a few similarities in the conceptual rationales of Rosabeth Kanter and June Holley.[2]

If we are satisfied that the type of coordinator role we have described—the characteristics it requires and the rationale informing it—is feasible in informal and formal networks of individuals and organizations, we have not yet been given those kinds of descriptions and analyses that would be of practical import for the relationship between rationale and practice. The accounts of Kanter and Holley gloss over the phenomenology and actions of those engaged in the process, so that the reader inclined to initiate and engage in the process has no guidelines for action.

In Holley's case, the omission is deliberate. There is "no one right way," she writes, and "attempts to help one community replicate another community's programs are likely to fail. . . . What communities need is not a blueprint, but the skills and understanding that will enable them to create their own field of possibilities." One cannot take exception to that statement. But, concretely, how did Holley decide to start where she did in the ways that she did? It would be useful for us to look at this as part of our developing an approach for other communities, but we are not told.

Holley also recommends caution in the use of measures of sustainability, as evaluation tools tend to make people think in terms of "discrete bits"—the aspects of the program that can be measured—rather than in global terms and thus tend to limit experimentation and exploration. "As an alternative," the report says,

> We suggest an emphasis on incorporating processes for reflection
> and continual improvement into community-based joint projects.
> In these processes, participants representing all of the stakeholders
> in the project are encouraged to analyze their work thus far, from
> quantitative, qualitative, and intuitive perspectives, and to identify
> what has worked well and how the project might be improved. At

the same time, the project's relationship to the larger systems of community and world are considered. Through these processes, basic evaluative skills that help individuals consider the community and worldwide impact of actions can be introduced. Screens and measures that emerge from these processes are likely to be more thoroughly internalized and thus have a far greater impact than those mandated up front by a local agency.

Again, concretely, what are these "processes of reflection"? Who was instrumental in initiating them, what are the characteristics of the processes or forums, what were the problems, how were they overcome? We offer these questions as a way of calling attention to what we need to know and learn, both from successes and failures. This sort of lapse is what has long concerned us in reports about conventional and unconventional coordinator roles. It is not a concern peculiar to this particular activity. You can write the history of science from the standpoint of how incomplete description of research procedures has had untoward, negative consequences. In the case of June Holley's work, we are not questioning outcomes. But if we are truly to capitalize on the accomplishments of Holley and her colleagues, we need to know more than we have been told. Fairness requires us to say that that kind of descriptive knowledge should not be expected from practitioners, i.e., from someone like Holley who spends her days and a good deal of her nights in action. It is amazing she has written as much as she has and that it is as seminal as it is. But it should be the obligation of policymakers and researchers in this area to get the details for us because there are many implications of her work for theory and practice.

Helping Those Who Help Themselves

We turn now to another example, the Industrial Areas Foundation (IAF). The IAF was created fifty years ago by Saul Alinsky, who is legendary in the arena of community organizing for the purpose of empowering poor and unlistened-to segments of a community to help themselves, i.e., to be able to contact, influence, and alter their relationship to the political system and the private sector. It is beyond our purpose to describe in detail how IAF works and the results its members have helped achieve; there is quite a literature on IAF (Horwitt, 1992; Rogers, 1990; Industrial Areas Foundation, n.d.). What is of importance are some of the similarities between our rationale and that of IAF. Our languages and labels are different, as are our organizational processes, but there are several features clearly in common. The first is that you cannot be helpful to people who are resigned to a stance of helplessness, a stance that permits them to see any alteration in their lives as having to come from somewhere "out there." They see themselves as without assets, influence, and power. They are aware only of their deficits, their lacks. IAF does not come on the scene unless some group in that community (usually a group of churches) invites them to come and is able to provide funds to support an "organizer" for two years.[3]

The second similarity, a partial one, is in the organizer's role. The IAF organizer does not fit the conventional notion of an organizer. He or she does not come with a predetermined agenda, nor expect to become a leader on the spot. Instead, the organizer uses the budget provided by the sponsoring committee to *talk*: to hold hundreds of one-on-one meetings with people in the community, building a comprehensive picture of the formal and informal networks of leadership, the community concerns, and the issues that will bring people together. Once that picture reaches a workable level of clarity, the organizer begins to convene small groups of eight to a dozen people, encouraging the participants to get to know each other and to decide to do something about some issue of mutual concern—not necessarily the biggest and most important issue, but one that the group can get a grip on and use to make a difference in their own lives. The organizer's role in these meetings is not to *organize*, i.e., to select goals and assign tasks, but rather to encourage the emergence of local leaders and to teach people how to organize themselves, with a view to extending their vision beyond immediate local concerns. The organizer is a listener, a total scout, a goad who does not see people through a prism for deficits but rather one for assets. The immediate goal is not to do something about this or that community action or issue but rather to promote attitudes and self-perceptions that counter feelings of hopelessness and resignation and begin building strengths.

This is exactly what we mean when we distinguish between prevention geared to a pathology and prevention that promotes capacities and well-being. The organizer does not accept responsibility for a course of action. If he or she has done the job well, responsibility is willingly accepted by the community participants.

Here is an example of one such program in action, a school project initiated by Dr. Paul Heckman of the University of Arizona. It is an attempt to alter schools in the poorest (Hispanic) sections of the city, and to do so by drawing on parents and community agencies, those with a stake in the schools. Sarason, who has had the good fortune to be associated with this program for the last five years, writes:

> At the first meeting I attended I was struck by the heterogeneity among the participants, ranging from individuals whose speech I had difficulty comprehending to those, mostly affiliated with local churches, who were obviously well educated in the conventional sense. I was also struck by their stance: they were not coming hat-in-hand to ask for help from a university-based project. They had been invited to the meeting and what they sought was clarification of a basis that would be mutually enhancing both to community needs, which went far beyond school improvement, and the school project. There were no confrontations. It was a discussion centering around how the resources of each party could be interconnected, i.e., how the resources of each could be increased.
>
> In previous years, I had been involved in scores of meetings among parents, community agencies, and school personnel. In all such meetings the stance of the educators was: "Here is how we think you can be helpful to us." The stance of the other participants was: "Tell us how we can be helpful and we will see if and how we

can be helpful." At that first Tucson meeting it was refreshingly clear that whatever agreements emerged would not, could not, be of the one-way-street variety. That was not explicitly articulated, but it was what the conversation was all about.

That meeting—and the twenty such meetings I have attended since—was quite different. The sessions bear a strong resemblance to the meetings of my own Westchester network. The active, incisive, and creative participation of parents increased dramatically over the five-year period; they did not get bored and frustrated and drift away. The truly dramatic point of all this is that one of the participants—clearly a well-educated, very well-spoken Anglo—contributed only rarely to the discussions. It was obvious that he was totally attentive to what was being said but he was silent for the most part. He never, so to speak, carried the ball. Others from the community did so. The silent participant was Frank Pearson, the IAF organizer. He had done his job extraordinarily well [Sarason, 1992].

The effect of the IAF on emerging local leaders is electric. A member of the San Antonio Communities Organized for Public Service (COPS) told an interviewer:

I got out of the house when I joined COPS. It was like a whole new world. I never knew I had so many talents. In 1982, I was elected area vice president. One of my first actions was to go before the city council to demand [to know] where money allocated for our neighborhood had gone. Christine, the organizer, coached me. We did a lot of research. There was $300,000 allocated for Amistad, and the money was moved elsewhere. We formed a committee and met with our city council representative and then the head of Community Development Block Grants. We demanded to see the notes of a meeting when the money was discussed. We learned that it was moved to another part of the city as a loan and we could not demand it back. I always remember the day we went to city council. My throat was dry, my legs were shaking. I was petrified. Just before

I started to speak, I turned around. There were 40 leaders from my parish behind me. I'll never forget that. That is the strength we have [Watriss, 1990].

A member of Valley Interfaith in South Texas told the same interviewer:

People in the Valley had been taught to understand that the system was only supposed to work for a few. People were passive. In the men's class I attended at my church, I was watching the same problems go on and on. I didn't see why my people had to get help through cheese lines—waiting, sometimes two to three hours in the sun, to get five pounds of cheese and some canned goods. It was embarrassing, insulting, and I became angry—an anger that makes you want to struggle against those who don't understand. . . . It's been real growth for me. I couldn't stand in front of people and talk when I started. Now I have been on stage in front of 5,000 and 10,000 people. When I see these people, I am energized. I see through their eyes that I am growing. Seven years ago, I never would have thought that one day I would be in Washington talking to one of the Congressmen. It is a "university of the people"—that's what we call our organization in the Valley. At this point, I don't know where or when to stop.

The practical goal of IAF is to relate to the private sector and the political system in ways that speak to the self-interests of all. They have done so and are doing it with a minimum of open conflict or resort to naked power. Their power resides in several things, two of which deserve emphasis. The first is that the community does its homework, i.e., people do what IAF calls "research," which gives them the data and knowledge to establish their credentials when they meet with private-sector or political figures. They do not come to these meetings asking for justice and fairness in the abstract. They come with concrete data about concrete issues and with concrete proposals, and they are prepared to participate in and accept responsibilities for implementation.

Geoffrey Rips, a former editor of the *Texas Observer*, put it this way:

> What we have in the Texas IAF Network is a great experiment. Can a meaningful relationship be developed between a politics based upon moral understanding and moral imperatives and the big-money politics of the late twentieth century? Is there still room to think and to build based upon values? Can a political system in which most people feel powerless be made a means of empowerment?
>
> As Ed Chambers described it, the source of IAF's strength is the relationship among individuals. "All of us have pain and joy in our lives. Once you hear it from a white person or a black person or a Mexicano, a Puerto Rican or a Latino, you say, gee, that's my story. That's the same story. We've got something in common. Once that starts happening to you, then you have a bond that the received culture doesn't put any value on. That's what keeps you together—your shared stories and your shared memories. That will keep you together and carry you through."
>
> Czech writer Milan Kundera once equated "the struggle of man against power" [meaning the State] with the "struggle of memory against forgetting." The politics of Texas IAF are the politics of the long haul. Communities are built upon collective memory, just as modern-day politics depend upon collective amnesia. The convention of the Texas IAF Network was an attempt to meld the politics of memory into a relationship with the politics of forgetfulness. It was awkward, but it worked. And to the extent that it continues to work, democracy is served [Geoffrey Rips, personal communication].

Nothing that the IAF has accomplished is understandable (or replicable) unless one grasps its bedrock assumption that you build on strengths, on assets real or potential, a building that requires methods or processes by which people use and "trade" those assets for very practical purposes. The assumption is what our description of a resource exchange is based on, an assumption implicit in the new paradigm of modern organization.

Notes

1. The discussion in this section is based in large part on a long paper by June Holley and Amy Borgstrom, titled "Growing Sustainable Communities." It spells out a comprehensive rationale that is as conceptually impressive and sophisticated as any we have read, without the underlying shallowness often found in such documents. Readers can obtain copies of this unpublished paper by writing to Holley at ACEnet, 94 North Columbus Rd., Athens OH 45701.

2. When we entertain the fantasy that if Rosabeth Kanter and June Holley were to sit in the same room with Mrs. Dewar and Daphne Krause, we believe the four would disagree about little. We offer, obviously thinking it is worth something, the observation that with rare exceptions, in our experience those who have the characteristics of the type of coordinator we have described are women.

3. The IAF has had little to do with schools in the past, but in recent years it has become aware that success in community organizing requires work in the schools. Unless schools become more sensitive to, knowledgeable about, and better coordinated with their social surrounds, they will not contribute, except in the most superficial ways, to the enhancement of community resources. Professor Dennis Shirley of Rice University has very well described this new direction. He kindly sent us a draft manuscript (Shirley, n.d.) of a book titled *Laboratories of Democracy: Building Political Power in Urban Schools and Neighborhoods.* We found the manuscript both instructive and compelling, and we look forward to its publication.

Epilogue: The Public Schools and the Private Sector

Whatever happens in our schools, especially in our urban areas, will be fateful for our society. More specifically, if the inadequacies of our schools continue or get worse, which is not unlikely, they will have increasingly destabilizing effects on our society. As we have repeatedly noted, schools are not unique organizations. They are different, but in terms of organizational rationale they have features very similar to those in private organizations or in government—features that have been subjected to criticism in those contexts with useful results. The products of industry are not the products of schooling, but the inadequacies of both that became so obvious after World War II have in principle highly similar causes, similarities that neither side has often been able to see or comprehend. As we shall soon see, the continued failure to note these similarities in their historical contexts will have untoward effects both on schools and the private sector. If, as we indicated in earlier chapters, some adaptive changes have begun to take place in the private sector (and we do not want to exaggerate the extent of change), the same is not true for schools. They have, generally speaking, been intractable to change (Sarason, 1990) despite many different types of efforts and the expenditure of billions of dollars, one result of which is general agreement that whatever the causes the answer is not to spend more money. To return to our recurring maxim, when we are faced with an intractable problem, it is a surefire sign that there is something very wrong or missing in the way we think.

Signs of Hope

The inadequacies of schools have been recognized, and their intractability is no less obvious. Nevertheless, we have elsewhere (Sarason, 1994) described exceptions that are instructive precisely because they are grounded on a concept of prevention that starts not with the deficits of students but with their strengths, not with correcting deficits but with expanding students' interests and experience. Indeed, it was this preventive orientation that in its early history propelled the Northern Westchester Network to use schools as a means of implementing and testing the resource exchange rationale. In earlier chapters, we have described instances of how productive that effort was. It was possible only because it successfully interconnected schools with a host of individuals and agencies (not only local) having something to contribute to and get from those interconnections. In short, boundary crossing increased the resources of all participants, not only students.

A more recent and truly exciting example is the accelerated schools program of Henry Levin (1993). Let us listen to Levin's account of the transformation in his thinking (summarizing would be an injustice):[1]

> The ideas for the accelerated school had their origin in work that I did in the late sixties and in the seventies on urban schools. . . . Up until the early eighties, I limited my research to the outer workings of schools, evaluating the financing arrangements, organizational incentives, and other external conditions affecting their success. I avoided the inner workings—that is, the details of teaching and learning. As an economist specializing in the economics of education, I saw curriculum and instructional strategies as being beyond the purview of my expertise.
>
> All of this changed in the eighties, when I was confronted with the plethora of national reports calling for educational reform for college-bound youngsters. These reports said nothing about students in at-risk situations with high dropout rates or the improve-

ment of elementary schools. I was struck by the absence of concern for those populations for whom we had dedicated the War on Poverty.

Curiosity led me to inquire into what had happened to so-called disadvantaged or at-risk student populations. I found that the national reports omitted them for matters of convenience, not for lack of severity of their situation. Sadly, the War on Poverty had not been won when it came to these children. By 1984 I had prepared a demographic study for Public/Private Ventures in Philadelphia, which showed that these students were a large and increasing portion of the student population and were still at great risk of school failures. Moreover, I found that existing educational reforms were unlikely to do much for these students, because the reforms focused primarily on raising high school standards for college-bound students rather than on improving the preparation of students who were dropping out under existing standards.

At this point, I plunged into a study of the internal practices of schools attended by at-risk students. I buried myself in the Cubberley Library at Stanford University to review reams of research on at-risk students and school practices as well as evaluations of purportedly effective programs. I undertook scores of interviews with teachers, parents, principals, central office administrators, state and federal education authorities, and academics with expertise on the subject. Finally, I visited schools around the country with high concentrations of at-risk students to observe existing practices.

From these activities, I came to a startling conclusion: the inevitable consequences of existing educational practices used with students in at-risk situations actually undermined the future success of these students. Even though these students started school behind other students in academic skills, they were placed in instructional situations that slowed down their progress. They were stigmatized as remedial students or slow learners and assigned boring and repetitive exercises on worksheets. Their parents were often uninvolved in the school, and school staff were given little or no opportunity to provide more challenging and successful approaches. School districts, with the support of the publishers, had saddled schools with "teacher-proof" approaches that consisted of low-level textbooks in combination with student workbooks full of dull and tedious exercises. Rarely did I see opportunities for problem solving, enrichment, or applications of knowledge that drew upon student experiences and interests.

To me the solution seemed obvious: instead of slowing down these students—with the inevitable consequence of getting them farther and farther behind—we needed to *accelerate* their progress to bring them into the educational mainstream. Accordingly, I drew on research on learning and effective organizations to design and implement a process whereby schools could accelerate the learning of students in at-risk situations. It became clear that schools implementing such a process would have to draw on the talents of all of their staff, students, and parents and would have to be based on effective approaches to gathering information, making decisions, and building incentives for success at all levels. Finally, I found the appropriate learning approach in the enrichment strategies used for gifted and talented students—the design of creative approaches that build on strengths. . . .

Accelerated schools represent an attempt to create schools that deepen the learning of all students, bring them into the educational mainstream by the end of elementary school, and continue that advancement in middle school and beyond. The full transformation of a school takes five or six years, but there are major gains even in the first year. An important goal of the Accelerated Schools Project is to provide the best educational and life options for *all* students while also clearly reducing the dropout rate, drug use, and the number of teenage pregnancies in secondary schools as a by-product.

Accelerated schools are built on a unity of purpose among the entire school community in creating practices and activities that are dedicated toward accelerated progress. They establish an active school-site decision-making process with responsibility for results, and active participation in decisions by all school staffs as well as

parents, with reliance on small-group task forces, a schoolwide steer-
ing committee, and schoolwide governance groups. Instead of focusing on weaknesses, accelerated school staff and parents use a
pedagogy constructed on the strengths and cultures of the children
(and indeed all members of the school community), with a heavy
reliance on relevant applications, problem solving, and active and
"hands-on" learning approaches as well as an emphasis on thematic
learning that integrates a variety of subjects into a common set of
themes. Finally, parental involvement both at home and at school
is central to the success of an accelerated school [Levin, 1993].

The *Resource Guide* from which that extended excerpt is taken
is an unusually comprehensive statement of rationale and process.
As Levin indicates, the rationale and process are no quick fix; they
require at the outset the realization that one has embarked on a
venture of literally "reinventing" schools. Nothing will remain the
same. Levin is not tinkering.

History and Ahistory

In one important respect, this epilogue contradicts our previous
point that only in recent decades have organizational theorists and
practitioners begun dramatically to alter their views about coordination, resource exchange, and structure in formal organizations.
The point is true for those in and around the private sector. It is
certainly *not* true in regard to our public schools, as we shall
endeavor to describe. Why this has not been recognized by organizational theorists and practitioners is an important part of the story
because the lack of recognition speaks volumes about boundary
crossing in regard to knowledge and experience.

It is probably still the case today that no school of business,
administration, or management has in its program anything about
public education that could be dignified as respectable in terms
of scholarship and research. The same judgment holds *within* the

university for the relationship between those schools and the school of education. (Yale, for example, has a school of organization and management. It has neither a school nor a department of education.)

It would require a separate book to examine this issue and its consequences in detail, but it is useful to sketch or outline the story. We assume that no reader of this book is unaware that today the private sector is concerned with the public schools, really anxious about their adequacy, and concerned and anxious as never before that the health of the private sector and social fabric is at risk. Put another way, unlike the concern felt in earlier decades, this concern goes beyond narrow, self-serving interests. Ironically, the executives who voice this concern rarely have any idea how influential the private sector was in forming the structure and organization of public schools; nor do they see why the public schools, unlike the private sector, have changed little if at all in response to changing circumstances.

The structure and organization of the public schools as we know them today is a direct descendant of what they became in response to waves of immigration in the nineteenth century and the early decades of the twentieth century. It was not unusual for classrooms then to have fifty or sixty children—or more. Not only were classrooms highly regimented, but so was the school and the school system, which steadily increased in the number of parts as well as the number of managers and administrators. Coordination of those parts was justified in terms of efficiency—which meant two things. First, cohorts of children would move smoothly from one grade to another (the grade structure became more and more differentiated) and from a lower school to a higher one. When it became apparent that some (not a few) students appeared not to have the ability (social, intellectual, or physical) to adjust to classroom requirements (i.e., they interfered with efficiency), new "parts" or programs were added to deal with them. If students dropped out of school, almost regardless of age or grade, there was a "part" to find them—but the number of such students was truly so large that for all practical purposes many remained out of the school system. Second, in practice, efficiency meant that each part of the organization did its own thing; it did not mean that parts were coordinated in any meaningful way, i.e., as long as each part took care of its assigned chores and did not interfere with other parts or present problems to them, coordination in the service of the system's goals would be achieved. When the inevitable problems occurred (caused by the organization chart mentality), the response was to create a new part with new administrative personnel. The organization charts changed frequently, taking on a complexity that the charts depicted as efficient and coordinated. The reality was quite otherwise.

Those were the days when factories were getting larger and larger, the concept of the assembly line was taking hold, and efficiency and coordination were paramount issues. It was not surprising that Henry Ford became a hero; his genius in organizing a coordinated mode of production was much acclaimed. His influence, and that of others like him, went beyond the private sector and became part of the imagery and thinking of those in public education who were struggling, especially in urban areas, to cope with their ever-growing, problem-producing educational "factories." Needless to say, there were more than a few industrial tycoons who were critical of public schools for ill preparing students to work in their factories; their criticisms were directed at school personnel for an impractical curriculum and poor leadership and administration. This was akin to the criticism that the very male Professor Henry Higgins in Shaw's *Pygmalion* (later *My Fair Lady*) directed to women: Why can't they be like us? If there were some educators who resented those criticisms, the fact was that city schools and school systems *did* bear resemblance to factories. In those early days this was not true for rural areas, where there were one-room schoolhouses (or very small schools) with all of the features of the "undermanned setting" so well described and conceptualized by Barker and Gump (1964). Those features, ironically, are very similar to the ones advocated by today's critics of traditional organizational structure. It is unfortunate but not surprising that Barker's book (1968) and other writings of his are never cited in the organizational literature. This is not surprising because the ethos and structure of the university are mammoth obstacles to the coordination and application of knowledge. Of course, if you examine the organization chart of a university, it is a coordinated structure of parts; but they are independent parts, frequently alien to each other. Their knowledge is compartmentalized, and therefore its potential for "added value" on the basis of a principle akin to resource exchange is blunted. This is also frequently the case *within* a part such as a department.

Let us assume, however, that there had been no relationship whatsoever between what happened in the industrial sector and the public schools. Nevertheless, they had one thing in common that would have produced what each became. We refer to a way of thinking consisting of three related views of people:

1. Whatever people were or could be—whatever their interests, curiosities, knowledge, and goals—was irrelevant to their assigned task in the workplace. They were laborers and not workers; that is, to some extent at least, workers put a personal imprint on a product, while laborers did not.

2. It was not the obligation of the overseers to be sensitive to, capitalize on, and employ the individuality of those they supervised. It was their obligation to see that people in the work setting conformed to the requirements of the narrow task assigned to them.

3. In these settings, people were a kind of human clay to be molded according to predetermined specifications. If they could not shape up, they were shipped out.

The National Park Service display of employee life in mills and factories in New England provides vivid confirmation of these points. (It is in Lowell, Massachusetts, and is well worth a visit.)

Henry Ford later paid his workers more—but the culture of his work site was no different. The urban schools, where immigrant children were explicitly objects of a taming and socializing process, were the direct equivalent of those mills and factories. That the purpose of schooling had fundamentally anything to do with *individuality* was a foreign idea. Not even foreign: it was inconceivable, never up for discussion in schools. With very rare exceptions, if anything captures the ambience of those schools, it is the word *impersonal.*[2]

Given their conception of people, their rapid growth and their fondness for efficiency, and the general conception of citizenship that made the taming and socialization process both necessary and desirable, schools would have become factories independent of what was happening in American industry. What the latter contributed was pressure to produce workers, plus the wonders and imagery of the coordinated assembly line. What schools became was overdetermined.

In this book, we have described a new paradigm for the relationship between organizational structure and a conception of people, a change having radical implications about what coordination should mean. The vaunted efficiency depicted in the organization chart has begun (and it has *only* begun) to be replaced by an imputed messiness reflecting a different conception of what people are and can be, of what an organization has to do if it is successfully to cope with fast, technology-stimulated change, of the need for boundary crossing to replace the one person, one function mode of organizational living.

We do not expect the advocates of this change to be knowledgeable about why schools became what they were and still are. The ahistorical stance is alive and well—unfortunately. So when some very well-intentioned corporate leaders grow alarmed at the inadequacies of our schools, their recommendations for reform essentially leave untouched the ethos of and rationale for the governance structure of schools that, historically, the private sector itself had mightily influenced. They call for reduction or elimination of "bloated bureaucracies," a greater emphasis on "basics," a strengthening of adherence to traditional standards of performance, judgments that face up to the results of cost-benefit analyses, and a greater imaginativeness that would make classroom learning more interesting and productive. Someone said it is hard to be completely wrong, and that holds for these critics. What they totally ignore is that the rationale for the governance structure of schools is still the rationale of earlier days. Schools are not the "factories" they once were, but their underlying social-psychological rationale continues to have similarly stultifying effects on students, teachers, principals, and others (Sarason, 1995b). The governance structure of schools has changed not at all, for practical purposes; where it has changed, this confirms the maxim that the more things change the more they remain the same.

Prefiguring the New Paradigm

The critics display equal ignorance of the fact that at the same time schools were taking on their still-current shape and features, a number of educators were already viewing those features as disasters. In fact, foremost among them was one person whose corpus of writings contains almost all of the ingredients today's organizational theorists advocate—and whose proposals some private-sector organizations have taken seriously. More than that, his writings, beginning a hundred years ago, continued over the decades to be influential in the thinking and actions of small groups of educators whose demonstrations have had no impact on schools generally. The point we are here making is that there have always been people on the educational scene who understood well that as long as schools employed a rationale for governance structure that aped that of the private sector, schools would be grossly inefficient, morally indefensible, and ultimately one of the most potent contributors to social destabilization.

We are referring to John Dewey: psychologist, philosopher, educator, social critic, visionary. His voluminous writings defy summary—any attempt would require a far-from-small book. We must be content with a series of bare-bones statements most relevant to our purposes. In so proceeding, we do not want to convey the impression that his writings contain a "theory of organizational structure" or that they speak in a direct way to the problems of coordination—though Dewey was a scathing critic of the presumed glories of efficient coordination in the private sector.[3] Dewey in no way fits the picture of the armchair theoretician and philosopher. He did enunciate principles and a point of view that were flatly and explicitly opposed to what schools were becoming, principles that in fact were manifest in the laboratory school he created at the University of Chicago at the end of the nineteenth century:

- *From their earliest days children are curious, questing, questioning, exploring organisms.* When they start school, they are not mindless, unorganized characters without awe and wonder about themselves, others, and the world. They are already budding scientists and artists.

- *The classroom should be a place where children's constructive characteristics are recognized and respected.* To put it negatively, one does *not* start with a predetermined curriculum that ignores individuality and from the start requires the child to set aside what is in his or her mind, instead to conform, to learn what grownups think he or she needs. If you do not start with where children are, you are beginning the process of extinguishing motivation for and interest in what society wants children to learn.

- *Children have assets for productive learning.* They have strengths, and you build on them. If they are viewed as empty vessels or as deficit-ridden—as organisms to be "filled" and deficits to be repaired—you will more often than not end up blaming the victim, i.e., proving you were right in the first place.

- *Schools are not preparation for life; they are life itself.* The classroom is a place where almost all the values and problems of life in a democracy come up, and if they are not discussed and reflected in teacher-student and student-student relationships, in how the classroom is structured and run, in its "constitution," then the children and the society are shortchanged. If you regard students as in dire need of taming and socialization, as if they are incapable of understanding and insensitive to the complexities of democratic living, then schools will be factories, production machines, a mockery of the democratic ethos.

It should be obvious from these points why Dewey was so critical of schools for their view of children, and critical of a school structure whose main "virtue" was to prepare students to take the role of ciphers in industry. No one needed to tell Dewey that industry was organized on the assumption that workers had no minds—besides which, if they had minds, they had better leave them at home. Dewey was not a fan of Henry Ford's. More than anyone else of his time, he sought to protect the child's "life of the mind." He saw that the way industry viewed people and the way it was organized came with a high price and that someday that price would be seen as self-defeating. He was, of course, right.

Let us now continue with more of Dewey's position.

- *Teachers should not be "commanders" (Dewey's word) embodying the executive, legislative, and judicial branches of classroom government.* The central point was that commanders tell people what to do and how to do it; they are the fount of knowledge from which pours information and facts to be memorized. That was the polar opposite of the context that makes for productive learning. Filling empty vessels with facts should never be confused with communicating with active minds about what they know and want to know.

- *The role of the teacher is one of coaching, managing, and arranging the learning environment.* This role appears messy in contrast to one where the teacher is essentially a well-meaning autocrat. It is a role ever sensitive to individual and group needs and changes, i.e., unpredictability is to be expected and not to be seen as interference with routine.

- *It is the obligation of the teacher to establish a relationship with parents.* Teachers need to realize that a parent has knowledge, is an asset, and has rights that should be respected. Parents are not foreign intruders but part of the enterprise. They can be valuable assets—but not if you see them as "just" parents.

- *Teacher-teacher and teacher-administrator relationships need to reflect the same mutual respect and attentiveness as teacher-student and teacher-parent relationships.* Dewey saw all of these relationships as generally lacking the features that make learning and growth more than a sometime thing. He regarded his psychological rationale for productive development in children to be totally applicable, morally and intellectually, to all stakeholders in the educational scene.

- *A school and school system exist in a community.* The community contains human and material resources about which school personnel *and* students should have working knowledge so that those resources can be tapped for educational purposes. The boundaries between school and society should be porous. The more schools are encapsulated places—the more the individual classroom is isolated from the rest of the school—the more completely potential resources remain just that: potential, unmined, unconnected to the education of children.

If Dewey did not give us anything like a systematic conception of how a school should be organized, he did give us a psychological and moral rationale for human relationships in any organization. If he did not want schools to be factories, he also did not want *factories* to be factories where human resources were ignored and underused. It is impossible to read Dewey and ignore that whatever he said about children, teachers, administrators, parents, and communities he regarded as no less applicable and valid for the workplace. Dewey was crystal clear about the difference between laboring and working, between mindless routine and personal expression, between being treated as ciphers and possessing assets, between derogation and respect, between tunnel vision and expansion of horizons. If Vice President Gore's reports on reinventing government had been published a hundred years ago, their psychological and moral rationale would have been scathingly criticized for "Deweyism."

Neither Dewey nor his critics, then and now, were in doubt that what he stood for was a radical transformation of what public and private organizations were and still largely are. That Dewey, so to speak, put his money where his mouth was can be seen in Mayhew and Edwards's (1966) description of his laboratory school at the University of Chicago. Coordination, boundary crossing, resource exchange, redefinition of resources, employment and interconnectedness of external resources—those concepts or labels are not to be found in the detailed description, but they clearly are reflected in it. Compared to schools of the time, Dewey's school was indeed messy; depicting its structure and purposes in an organization chart would be about as revealing as a restaurant menu is to the food served. Dewey was no organizational theorist. To regard him as such would be an egregious example of reading the present into the past. But it would be no less egregious to continue to ignore the direct relevance of what he wrote and did to life in organizations. Aside from being a psychologist, philosopher, educator, and logician, he was a most penetrating social observer and critic. His interests went far beyond the schools.

International Comparisons

Today we are constantly reminded, especially by private-sector executives (for obvious reasons), that Japanese schools are far more effective than ours. By conventional criteria for academic performance, they clearly are more effective. The critics point to differences like these: the Japanese school year is longer, the "basics" are emphasized, the quality of teachers and teaching is better even though the average Japanese classroom has more children than the American one, and standards are high and adhered to. Why cannot our schools be like theirs? (We are back to Henry Higgins!) At the same time, the American private sector has been criticized for its styles of organizational structure and management, which have rendered it relatively uncompetitive with the Japanese private sector. Soon after Japan's defeat in World War II, Japanese industry was mightily influenced and transformed by W. Edwards Deming's concept of Total Quality Management (TQM). The critics of American industry seem never to have noted the startling similarities between Deming's psychological and moral rationale and Dewey's. Even those educators who have seen the relevance of TQM for the American classroom have not noted its kinship to Dewey.

Early in this century, Dewey was invited to China and Japan to visit and observe schools and make recommendations for their improvement. In 1992 a Japanese educator, Manabu Sato, wrote the following:

> The progressive education era, 1947–1955, was the most vital one for teachers in the history of Japanese education. Child-centered education was a symbol of democratic society in the postwar age, and *Dewey's philosophy was the bible of almost every teacher.* The curriculum development movement, in which numerous teachers passionately participated, spread all over the country as the revitalization of the heritage of progressive education in the 1920s. Indeed, the national survey of the National Institute for Educational Research in 1951 indicated that over 80 percent of teachers participated in developing their own school curricula and that about 85 percent of the schools adopted the unit teaching method in social studies and in science teaching based on the doctrine of

child-centeredness. The movement led to professional autonomy, and teachers organized innumerable voluntary study groups both inside and outside of the schools. The Japan Teachers' Union, established in 1947, also enhanced teachers' autonomy by promoting voluntary studies. The union held annual study meetings for teachers at national, prefectural, and local levels, in which teachers developed their professional culture by sharing their practical experience and principles with each other [p. 161; italics added].

Although in no way a comprehensive explanation of the academic performance of Japanese students, this quotation has twofold significance for our discussion. First, it describes aspects of the culture of schools that are the polar opposite of those in America, where the potential assets of teachers (and administrators, for that matter) stand no chance of being recognized or applied, from their earliest socialization in preparatory programs onward (Sarason, 1993b). The Japanese school comes closer in its formal and informal aspects to Dewey's school than almost all of the hundreds of American schools we have personally seen. Second, the relationship among teachers is mirrored in their relationships with students and in the relationships among students. In brief, the "management style" reflects a psychological and moral rationale quite different from that in American schools. It is a style quite similar to the one that Deming advocated for Japanese industry, and that it bought, namely, a redefinition of workers as resources; boundary crossing; and a conception of coordination that emphasized more the informal than the customary formal, bureaucratically driven, mechanistic conception.

This point brings us to a startling implication (it is more than that) of something that Sato goes on to describe. As usual, the picture is more complicated and the grass is not so green as it looks on the other side; the preceding quote (and our comments) hold primarily for Japanese schools for the decade or so after the war, and apparently less so as time went on. Sato states: "The first symptom of this school crisis appeared as school violence broke out in 1980.

This spread particularly in junior high schools throughout the country year after year. After the wave of school violence had subsided, student apathy took its place. The newspapers, journals, and television news have reported increased numbers of dropouts, autistic children, juvenile delinquents, students with a psychological hatred of schooling, bullying children, teacher burnout, and their corporal punishment" (p. 157).

He also gives part (and only part) of the background:

The professionalization of teachers was aborted by revitalized bureaucratic policies beginning in the mid-1950s. Teacher freedom and autonomy were gradually restricted. First, teachers' political activities were prohibited by the Law Concerning Provisional Measures for Securing Political Neutrality of Education in Compulsory Schools and the revised Special Regulations for Educational Public Service Personnel in 1954. Second, the teacher's professional autonomy was also restricted. The national curriculum was announced in 1958, and the check system of textbooks was implemented. Since then, teachers have been obliged to be obedient to the national curriculum, which has been revised about every ten years. The textbooks, checked by the Ministry of Education, have become uniform. Even though teachers' salaries have been improved by governors, they were given in exchange for restricting their professional freedom and autonomy. . . .

What is more, teachers have become heavily burdened in coping with the pressures applied by parents and students under the entrance examination system and increasing student delinquency and apathy. In recent years, teachers have become isolated from one another because there is little time for interaction. . . .

Ten years from now, the teaching force will be occupied by the teachers who have been educated only in the bureaucratic, efficient schools. Informal functions to develop the teaching profession have become weak, and their priority for young teachers has diminished year by year. Instead, the formal functions of the teacher in-service training system have been strengthened [pp. 161–163].

We are not in a position to judge whether Sato is justified in suggesting that with the slow demise of Deweyan orientation in the face of an increasingly centralized bureaucracy, Japanese schools as they are now glowingly described will take on some of the negative aspects of American schools. Sato is *not* saying the Japanese schools lack the features they once had. The picture we get from Stevenson and Stigler (1991) is not invalidated; at the very least, unless Sato is grievously distorting the Japanese scene and its history since the war, he warns us that the organization chart mentality is likely changing schools in negative ways, a process to which Stevenson and Stigler may have been insensitive.

Dewey in America

Dewey's ideas never took hold in American schools. He had loads of advocates in our schools, but their rhetoric was belied by their practices. However, over the years there have been countless instances of *isolated* programs and demonstrations quite consistent with his ideas. We emphasize *isolated* because today we know of no public school, no "whole school," the organization and dynamics of which can be said to reflect Dewey's ideas.

The most notable (and best described) attempt to take Dewey seriously was the heroic "Eight Year Study," which concerned a sample of public high schools (Aiken, 1942). The study rested on as devastating a critique of schools generally, and high schools in particular, as has ever been written. It attempted to implement Deweyan ideas, and up to a point it did so successfully. Wonder of wonders, it even got three hundred colleges and universities to agree to admit students from these high schools other than by the usual criteria of grades and standard tests. It is beyond our purposes to say more about this study (done in the 1930s) except that it was far from a failure. Why did it have no impact? Was it because the report came out during World War II, when public education was not on the public agenda? Was it because what it advocated seemed to have messy implications for factorylike schools? Was it because the governance structure of schools (within a school and a school system) is based on a rationale that is totally inimical to risk taking, innovation, and apparent messiness? Whatever the combination of reasons, the fact is that with the cessation of the war high schools became larger, more bureaucratic, more stultifying than before.

It was not long after the war that the president of Harvard, James Conant, wrote his influential report on the comprehensive high school, a report that is a textbook case of the organization chart mentality running rampant. His report had all of the features of the presumed efficient coordination necessary in a large, differentiated organization. It contained none of the features of Dewey's psychological and moral rationale or, needless to say, the rationale for the private sector that *some* more recent theorists, consultants, and corporate leaders have advocated. Predictably, Conant's report was an invitation to continued disaster. His report, it should be noted, came at a time when the American private sector was operating on the myth that the future would be a carbon copy of the present: let us do more of the same! The auto industry, among others, was not prepared for its comeuppance. Neither were educators prepared for schools to become a cause for national anxiety and for educators themselves to be seen as inadequate, or insular, or self-serving, or unimaginative, or obstructing change. Or all of the above. It was (and is) a classic case of misplaced emphasis.

Let us return to the *organizational* implications of the nine statements given earlier about Dewey's viewpoint. The major implication derives from his emphasis that a classroom and a school should not be encapsulated from their surround. It should be the obligation of the school to be a meaningful part of the surround not only for purely educational purposes but for the ability to take advantage of the resources found there. The justification is that students should be exposed to the community and, additionally, you can count on students *wanting* to learn more about their surround. To underestimate that kind of wanting reflects a mammoth, inexcusable ignorance about people in general and students in particular. In addition, if anything characterizes young people it is the need to feel competent, to learn and do things in ways that bear their personal stamp and about which they have pride. They are also explorers.

None of these statements will strike a jarring note to the ears of the reader. These ideas are old hat. They were not old hat in Dewey's day, and anyone familiar with the vast literature on today's model American classroom would be justified in concluding that their application, at least, is not old hat today.

There are exceptions, of course. One of the most vivid involves the students of Shoreham-Wading River Middle School on Long Island in New York (Vlahakis, 1978). The program there rests on two foundations:

> First, it is necessary to have an administration that is concerned with providing teachers with an emotional and intellectual climate which encourages optimal learning conditions in the classroom. This means, among other things, shared decision-making. When there is an administrative climate that sustains, encourages, and provides opportunities for shared decision-making, success is more probable because the program reflects the values, experiences, and expertise of those who developed it.
>
> Secondly, the classroom should be a community in which students learn how to learn—learn to discover concepts, principles and generalizations that can be applied, through problem-solving, to the real problems of our civilization which defy the separation of "subject" approaches by their very complex nature. Knowledge, as Dewey noted, is external; knowing is internal. Certainly it is easier to be a disciple than an inquirer, but should not the schooling process be an active one in which students take an interest in their education, take responsibility for their learning, and consciously use knowledge to solve problems and understand relationships? [Silverblank, 1978, p. 1].

The results Vlahakis describes are indeed heartwarming. We have spent time at that school, and his description is consistent with our experience there. For our present purposes, we wish to emphasize several features of the school as prologue to a question we shall raise.

Most important, the principal of the school saw his primary obligations as enriching and enlarging the experience of everyone involved in the school. He devoted his attention to three efforts: (1) to stimulate and support teachers to be initiators, to support venturing in new directions even if success was by no means guaranteed, (2) to keep teachers, parents, and community people from regarding students (middle school youngsters) as "just" young kids incapable of assuming responsibility in a serious role, and instead to lead the community to expect more of the students beyond sitting in an encapsulated classroom in an encapsulated school, and (3) to gain access to individuals and sites in the surrounding community that could be exploited for the education of young people—and to help those community resources come to see the students as being helpful to them. This resource exchange is precisely what was accomplished, i.e., community sites benefited from the work of students, and students benefited mightily, intellectually and interpersonally, from being in those sites.

It could be argued (and was argued) that what happened there was possible because it had a Deweyan kind of principal, and, no less crucial, because it served a community of highly educated, "enlightened" parents willing to entertain and support Deweyan ideas (although the name of John Dewey, let alone his writings, was never in the picture). The same argument was advanced as a limiting factor in generalizing from Dewey's lab school: with unusual people you can do unusual things, but with others who are not like "us" it is another story. At its root, the argument is one that justified the factories of earlier times, i.e., you treated people according to their apparent limitations and deficits. For all practical purposes, they had no assets or strengths. (See Sarason, 1993a, for a more detailed discussion of these points.)

In the hundred-year interval between Dewey's lab school and Shoreham-Wading River Middle School, there have been countless demonstrations of what Dewey's ideas mean for organizational structure and ambiance, and for the transformations they imply and require. But these have all been isolated instances having no general impact whatsoever. The history of these ventures is totally unknown to contemporary theorists of organizational governance and some private-sector executives critical of schools. What they completely miss is how similar (not identical) the issues are in schools and private-sector *and* larger public organizations. We must emphasize, too, that they are ignorant of the long and sorry history of efforts to take Dewey's ideas seriously. So it is not surprising that in the documents justifying the vice president's goal of reinventing government—mightily influenced by so-called new ways of thinking about organizations—nowhere is there any recognition of the substance and history of the Deweyan rationale. Yet this is a government that has spent, and will continue to spend, billions upon billions of dollars to improve schools, in efforts that have failed in the past and—unless reinvented in ways similar in principle to those the vice president advocates for the federal government—will surely fail in the future.

The B.F. Day elementary school, once one of the worst schools in Seattle, offers another example of Dewey's philosophy in action (Quint, 1994). Although the principal probably was not familiar with Dewey's writings, it is as if she took seriously everything he advocated about what children (seen as people) are, can become, and can do if they are redefined as having assets and strengths. She had the willingness and courage to alter the structure and ethos of school and, in addition, the relationship of the school with countless individuals and agencies in its surround. Quint observes, "When the best elements of human nature rise above the oppressiveness of societal institutions, we can 'make each one of our schools an embryonic community life,' as John Dewey said a hundred years ago" (p. 124). The principal of the school was able to change its social climate and develop a philanthropic attitude and a new sense of purpose. She repudiated the existing "educational system as one which perpetuates the lifestyle patterns that prevail in a given community. She sought out social networks to transform her school into a multifaceted service agency committed to meeting the needs of the whole child and his or her family" (p. 125).

Quint obviously has a sense of history, which is more than can be said about many educators (and organizational theorists). It is, to say the least, refreshing to see John Dewey accorded recognition. Too often today, he is referred to pejoratively by critics of our schools who either never read Dewey or whose capacity to understand the printed word is truly meager.

We shall not attempt to summarize Quint's book, which we warmly recommend as further reading. Aspects of the rationale that suffused her account can be gleaned from one incident she describes. A local paraprofessional family support worker managed to find permanent housing for many of the families of homeless children attending B.F. Day elementary school. She did this by getting in touch with the landlord of a property infested with drug dealers and gang members, which the Seattle Times reported as facing a probable court-ordered closedown, and persuading him to allow homeless families to use apartments rendered vacant by eviction of undesirable tenants. Accepting the amount these new tenants could afford to pay (assisted in first-month deposits by a local fund) was far more beneficial to the landlord than leaving the property vacant and subject to vandalism; the apartments themselves, despite the building's unfortunate history, were far better for the new tenants than living on the streets. The initial contact with the landlord was through his lawyer, who attended the same church as the paraprofessional. When she got the landlord on the phone, she told Quint, "I just had to get him to agree, and so I kept talking until he could see that this was a mutually advantageous opportunity. That phone conversation was a major turning point." After thinking over the proposal, the landlord not only agreed but hired a homeless couple to serve as resident managers in the building. This couple—whom Quint describes at some length—took their job very seriously indeed, and settled in as managers in the old style, forming constructive attachments to the tenants, looking after children whose parents were temporarily absent, and even teaching people how to cook and otherwise take advantage of the facilities of a private apartment.

This was a living example of our oft-repeated motto of collaboration: "What do I have that somebody else can use in exchange for something of his that I need?" The landlord's lawyer was not part of the paraprofessional's immediate circle, but she had enough common ground with the lawyer to gain his help with the next step in the linkage. Had she not had the church contact, she could have found another. Mutual benefit speaks with a loud voice, once people allow themselves the freedom to stop and listen. As Quint points out, "If the school had still perceived itself as shackled to the bureaucracy, the apartment house would have gone empty, many children would not have had a caring adult to reassure them in the night, and two homeless, unemployed, but capable individuals would have had neither home nor jobs. By attending to realities that cried out for new solutions—solutions well beyond any stipulated in an official job description—the family support worker embraced the process of change and turned it into the process of achievement" (p. 81).

Quint's narrative would have warmed the cockles of Dewey's heart. Her book confirms everything we have said in previous chapters about coordination, resource exchange, and productive messiness. (Not so coincidentally, in 1989 the B.F. Day School ranked lowest among all sixty-five Seattle elementary schools in academic performance. Four years later, it was approaching the median, at thirty-eighth place.)

What specific bearing do these examples have for coordination and coordinators? We have stressed the point that coordination is not a matter of putting pieces together mechanistically. Resource exchange and boundary crossing powered by a resource exchange and network rationale requires coordinators who have the cognitive and personal characteristics discussed in Chapters Five and Six. Those requirements, we noted, have not received the attention they deserve, certainly not on a descriptive level. On that level, the Shoreham-Wading River example is more instructive, albeit incomplete in regard to coordinators' personal styles and how they were selected. But we are justified in several conclusions that are as applicable to schools as they are to private-sector organizations.

- It is not enough for the leader of the organization to grasp the rationale; he or she has to be a model *in action* of that rationale, just as Mrs. Dewar was in the informal Westchester network.

- If the leader models coordination, it makes it easier for others in the formal organization with "coordinator characteristics" to surface and be recognized. It also makes it more likely that the leader will choose coordinators who have the appropriate characteristics. (As noted in Chapter Five, it is dangerous to choose people simply because they want to be coordinators. It is necessary to be able to recognize those who can make a success of the job. That is why it is so important that the leader be the kind of coordinator he or she will have to select.)

- Having chosen a coordinator (or coordinators), the leader has to develop a forum where the issues of coordination are discussed, where one person learns from others, and where new possibilities for resource exchange or boundary crossing can be gleaned. Coordination is more than the achievement of a goal; it is a process of mining for resources within the organization and out into its community surround. It is a process that feeds on itself.

Conclusion

Finally, we return to a question we raised earlier in this book about private-sector organizations and the reinventing government effort, but now in relation to schools. Can the coordinating role be set up so that it does not get caught in the crossfire of power plays, which exist in schools as they do in other complicated organizations? In the Shoreham-Wading River instance, it was the principal and another administrator who enabled and ran interference for Mr. Vlahakis in locating community sites. He played a role, of course, but being a classroom teacher meant he did not have the time to do it by himself. Everyone in a school has full-time responsibilities, and it is asking too much to expect that they would have time to milk the potentials of the coordinating role; that holds too for the principal and others in administration. That limitation, however, loses force as, in the Seattle case, the rationale for boundary crossing not only transforms the school but attracts community people, some of whom are kin to Mrs. Dewar. Some of the most creative coordinators in the Seattle school were not formally part of the school, i.e., they had no formal power.

We raise these questions not because cumulative experience has provided answers but precisely because there is no such (published) experience and we wish to avoid conveying the impression that realizing the potential of the coordinating role is without organizational problems. It is not a matter of adding another box to the organization chart. We are identifying here issues for which there is a universe of alternatives to consider. There is no one answer. Of one thing we are sure: appropriately implementing the rationale for resource exchange and boundary crossing is not and should not be a simple affair. Viewing it as simple will only lead to one more confirmation of Mencken's caveat that for any complex problem there is a simple answer that is wrong. That maxim has already been confirmed zillions of times in the attempts to reform our schools and private-sector organizations.

Another confirmation may well be in progress. Not long ago, the city of Hartford gave over the running of its entire school system to a private, for-profit organization. This has been happening elsewhere on a less comprehensive basis. From what we know and have learned, the private company taking over the Hartford schools has a conception of efficiency and an organization chart mentality that force us to conclude that the venture will be the latest example of the predictable failure of educational reform.[4] There is nothing, but absolutely nothing, to suggest that this company has learned anything either from the history of education, from the writings of certain organizational theorists, or from the experience of corporate executives who unimprisoned themselves from longstanding conceptions of organizational rationale and structure. The city of Hartford's decision was an act of desperation. We are sure that the private company is well intentioned and "friendly" to the ostensible purposes of schooling. Unfortunately, with friends like that, educational decision makers need never worry about having enemies. Our schools today are a mess. Unlike the positive way we spoke about messiness in previous chapters, we mean the word here pejoratively. The stakes are too high for us to be circumspect in our criticism.

The points this Epilogue makes are best phrased in terms of questions. Why are schools so totally ignored by organizational theorists, and why are presumably new ways of thinking about organizational structure applicable only to the private sector? Why are the criticisms of schools by private-sector people based on the unverbalized assumption that the problems of resource exchange and boundary crossing are not as central or as intractable in schools as they are in private-sector organizations? Why even today are organizational theorists (let alone corporate executives) so ignorant of the fact that with the appearance of compulsory education in the nineteenth century, the structure and ambience of schools were those of industrial factories? (The similarity was noted and criticized by a man who offered a rationale that, if taken seriously, would have made for schools quite similar in important respects to what some respected organizational theorists are now advocating for the private sector.) Can one dispute the claim that what happens in and to the private sector in coming decades will be fateful for our society? Similarly, can one dispute the fact that what has happened to and in our schools in the post–World War II era—and what apparently will continue to happen—has been socially destabilizing and, we predict, will be more so in the future? Are we truly dealing with genotypically different entities?

We have provided some answers to these questions, although no one answer is comprehensive or can do justice to the complexities involved in answering them. We hope readers will continue to think about these questions, and to look at their own schools—the schools where they work, the schools their children attend, the schools in their communities—in the light these questions can shed on the quality and even the continuance of modern life.

Notes

1. Reprinted with permission of Dr. Henry Levin.
2. On the very day these words were first written (October 24, 1994), the front page of the *New York Times* had an article about an incipient parent insurrection in a Pennsylvania community following a proposal to double the population of the high school from eighteen hundred to thirty-six hundred students. New York City used to have schools as large or larger (it may still have). In earlier decades there would have been no reaction to such a proposal. Immigrant parents were seen as no different from their children, treated accordingly, and hardly heard from.
3. As the reader examines the statements to come, we urge keeping in mind that almost every one of them had, and largely still has, its *missing* counterpart in the rationale and structure of industrial organizations. It is quite a different story when these statements are compared to those that could be culled from the writings of Kanter and Holley described in Chapter Six, and those of Vice President Gore in Chapter One.
4. As this book was being completed, Hartford terminated the contract with the company, presumably for financial reasons. They are now asking the state to take over.

References

Aiken, W. A. (1942). *The story of the eight-year study with conclusions and recommendations*. New York: HarperCollins.

Albee, G. (1977, March). Some of my best friends are vegetarians. *Country Journal*, 62–67.

Barker, R. G., & Gump, P. V. (1964). *Big school, small school*. Stanford, CA: Stanford University Press.

Blumenkrantz, D. G. (1992). *Fulfilling the promise of children's services*. San Francisco: Jossey-Bass.

Freedman, M. (1993). *The kindness of strangers*. San Francisco: Jossey-Bass.

Frost, C. F., Wakeley, J., & Ruh, R. A. (1974). *The Scanlon plan for organization development, identity, participation, and equity*. East Lansing, MI: Michigan State University Press.

Gore, A. (1993a). *From red tape to results: Creating a government that works better and costs less*. Report of the National Performance Review. Washington, DC: Government Printing Office.

Gore, A. (1993b). *From red tape to results: Transforming organizational structures*. Report of the National Performance Review. Washington, DC: Government Printing Office.

Gore, A. (1993c). *From red tape to results: Strengthening the partnership in intergovernmental service delivery*. Report of the National Performance Review. Washington, DC: Government Printing Office.

Holley, J., & Borgstrom, A. "Growing sustainable communities." Unpublished manuscript, Appalachian Center for Economic Networks, Athens, OH.

Horwitt, S. D. (1992). *Let them call me rebel: Saul Alinsky, his life and legacy*. New York: Vintage Books.

Industrial Areas Foundation. *IAF: Fifty years of change*. IAF, 36 New Hyde Park Rd., Franklin Square, NY 11010.

Kanter, R. M. (1972). *Commitment and community: Communes and utopias in sociological perspective*. Cambridge, MA: Harvard University Press.

Kanter, R. M. (1994). Collaborative advantage: The art of alliances. *Harvard Business Review*, 96–108.

Kanter, R. M. (1995). *World class: Thriving locally in the global economy*. New York: Simon & Schuster.

Levin, H. (1993). Prologue. In W. Hopfenberg, H. Levin, & Associates (Eds.), *The accelerated schools: A resource guide*. San Francisco: Jossey-Bass.

Levine, M., & Levine, A. (1992). *Helping children: A social history*. New York: Oxford University Press. (Originally published in 1970 as *A Social History of Helping Services*.)

Lipnack, J., & Stamps, J. (1993). *The team net factor: Bringing the power of boundary crossing into the heart of your business*. Essex Junction, VT: Oliver Wight/Omneo.

Lipnack, J., & Stamps, J. (1994). *The age of the network*. Essex Junction, VT: Oliver Wight/Omneo.

Mayhew, K. C., & Edwards, A. C. (1966). *The Dewey school*. New York: Atherton Press.

National Council on Excellence in Education. (1983). *A nation at risk*. (Publication no. 065-000-00177-2). Washington, DC: Government Printing Office.

A 1996 National Education Summit Policy Statement. (1996, March). National Education Summit, Palisades, NY.

Norman, S. (1972).*The youth service bureau: A key to delinquency prevention*. Washington, DC: National Commission on Crime and Delinquency.

Quint, S. (1994). *Schooling homeless children: A working model for America's public school*. New York: Teachers College Press.

Rocawich, L. (1990, September). Ernesto Cortes, Jr.: Spark, challenge, agitate. *The Progressive*, 34–37.

Rogers, M. B. (1990). *Cold anger*. Denton, TX: University of North Texas Press.

Sarason, S. B. (1972). *The creation of settings and the future societies*. San Francisco: Jossey-Bass.

Sarason, S. B. (1990). *The predictable failure of educational reform: Can we change course before it's too late?* San Francisco: Jossey-Bass.

Sarason, S. B. (1993a). *Letters to a serious education president*. Thousand Oaks, CA: Corwin Press.

Sarason, S. B. (1993b). *The case for change: Rethinking the preparation of educators*. San Francisco: Jossey-Bass.

Sarason, S. B. (1994). *You are thinking of teaching? Opportunities, problems, realities*. San Francisco: Jossey-Bass.

Sarason, S. B. (1995a). *Parental involvement and the political principle:Why the existing governance structure of schools should be abolished*. San Francisco: Jossey-Bass.

Sarason, S. B. (1995b). *School change: The development of a personal point of view*. New York: Teachers College Press.

Sarason, S. B. (1996). *Revisiting the culture of the school and the problem of change*. New York: Teachers College Press.

Sarason, S. B., & Lorentz, E. (1989). *The challenge of the resource exchange network*. Cambridge, MA: Brookline Books. (Originally published in 1979.)

Sarason, S. B., & others. (1989). *Human services and resource networks*. Cambridge, MA: Brookline Books. (Originally published in 1977.)

Sato, M. (1992). Japan. In H. B. Leavitt (Ed.), *Issues and problems in teacher education: An international handbook*. Westport, CT: Greenwood Press.

Shirley, D. *Laboratories of democracy: Building political power in urban schools and neighborhoods*. Unpublished draft manuscript, Rice University.

Silverblank, F. (1978). Foreword. In R. Vlahakis, *Kids who care*. Oakdale, NY: Dowling College Press.

Stevenson, H. W., & Stigler, J. W. (1991). *The learning gap: Why our schools are failing and what can we learn from Japanese and Chinese education*. New York: Summit Books.

Thompson, V. L. (1985). *Adult learning in a resource exchange network: A case study of the Westchester resource exchange network*. Unpublished doctoral dissertation, Teachers College, Columbia University.

Towbin, A. P. (1978). The confiding relationship: A new paradigm. *Psychotherapy: Theory, Research, Practice, 15*(4).

Vlahakis, R. (1978). *Kids who care*. Oakdale, NY: Dowling College Press.

Watriss, W. (1990, November 22). Interview with Virginia Ramirez and Javier Parra. *Texas Observer*.

Index